About the authors

Richard Storey is a writer, photographer and a strong advocate of the life-changing potential of the Mount Athos Diet. He has personal knowledge of the Orthodox monastic life having for the past 15 years visited Mount Athos annually, both as a pilgrim and a voluntary worker. His photographic essay, *Images of Mount Athos*, was exhibited at Bridgewater House, London and at Highgrove House, Gloucestershire. Richard is an accomplished cook, trained in Classic French, Spanish, Indonesian, Thai and Modern British cookery. This is his fourth book.

Sue Todd is an editor who trained in nutrition, and through her career in food always aimed to help make healthy eating easier and more enjoyable. She has a degree in nutrition and worked as a State Registered Dietitian in the NHS in London for five years, before becoming the nutritionist at the consumer magazine, *Which?*. She then edited food websites for the BBC, UKTV and Carlton Food Network, and was Producer on BBC Radio 4's *Food Programme*. She was a trustee of the Caroline Walker Trust for over 10 years.

Lottie Storey is a writer who lives in Bristol with her husband and two young sons. Her work on the BBC Food website – recipe development, writing and proofing – contributed to the team winning the 'Best Interactive Media' Glenfiddich Food & Drink Award 2003 and an EMMA Award in 2002. In 2008 she founded a new branch of the Women's Institute. She has worked in publishing, digital marketing, PR, film, television, and the arts, and now writes full 'me, developing recipes and content for a range of client￼ g – oysterandpearl co.uk

This book is dedicated to

*The Holy Fathers of Mount Athos,
with gratitude for their inspiration.*

– Richard Storey

Eddy and Fenwick – Big love to you both.

– Sue Todd

*Ben, Arthur and Ted – Thank you for being
so patient and kind, and for overlooking the
mess in the kitchen. You are my world.*

– Lottie Storey

THE
MOUNT
ATHOS
DIET

THE MEDITERRANEAN PLAN
TO LOSE WEIGHT, LOOK
YOUNGER AND LIVE LONGER

By Richard Storey, Sue Todd and Lottie Storey

Vermilion
LONDON

1 3 5 7 9 10 8 6 4 2

Published in 2014 by Vermilion, an imprint of Ebury Publishing
Ebury Publishing is a Random House Group company

Copyright © Richard Storey, Sue Todd and Lottie Storey 2014

Richard Storey, Sue Todd and Lottie Storey have asserted their right
to be identified as the authors of this Work in accordance with the
Copyright, Designs and Patents Act 1988

The Random House Group Limited Reg. No. 954009

Addresses for companies within the Random House Group can be found at
www.randomhouse.co.uk

A CIP catalogue record for this book is available from the British Library

The Random House Group Limited supports The Forest Stewardship Council® (FSC®),
the leading international forest-certification organisation. Our books
carrying the FSC label are printed on FSC®-certified paper. FSC is the only
forest-certification scheme supported by the leading environmental organisations,
including Greenpeace. Our paper procurement policy can be found at
www.randomhouse.co.uk/environment

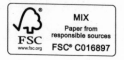

Designed and set by seagulls.net

Printed and bound by CPI Group (UK) Ltd, Croydon, CR0 4YY

ISBN 9780091954703

Copies are available at special rates for bulk orders.
Contact the sales development team on 020 7840 8487 for more information.

To buy books by your favourite authors and register for offers, visit
www.randomhouse.co.uk

CONTENTS

PREFACE

The Mount Athos Diet is a safe and easy-to-follow way to help you lose weight and look and feel a lot healthier. It does not involve any severe deprivation, or counting of calories. Nor will you have to buy special diet meals or drinks. All you will need to do is follow some straightforward principles and cook from a selection of delicious recipes. When you have reached your target weight, you should find it easy to maintain your new way of eating as well as your new weight and body shape.

HOW TO USE THIS BOOK

This book is structured in such a way that you can dip in and out of sections as you wish. You don't have to read it from cover to cover. Most readers will want to know 'what do I have to do?' and will turn immediately to the chapters concerned with the diet plan, recipes and ingredients. Whether you are vegetarian, a meat eater or vegan, there are plenty of recipes and advice to suit your lifestyle. Others will have questions about the background to the Mount Athos Diet: where does it come from, who else has tried it and what are their stories? There are further chapters devoted to exercise, drinking alcohol and meditation for readers who are interested in developing further aspects of their journey to a long-term way of eating and living a healthy life.

For further support and information, including beautiful images and more recipes, visit The Mount Athos Diet website: www.mountathosdiet.co.uk; find us on Facebook: www.facebook.com/themountathosdiet, or follow us on Twitter: www.twitter.com/mountathosdiet

A Word About Health

The Mount Athos Diet has been co-designed by a professional dietitian and its nutritionally balanced recipes will deliver a controlled and healthy weight loss. However, if you have any medical condition, are taking medication or are pregnant, breastfeeding or have an eating disorder, you should seek advice from your GP before starting any diet or exercise programme.

A Note On Ingredients

Unless specified, vegetables are peeled, and all ingredients should be the best quality available. Where possible, use organic or free-range eggs, dairy, meat and sustainable seafood.

HOW RICHARD 'DISCOVERED' THE MOUNT ATHOS DIET

I enjoy my food – and drink.

I have always been a gourmet (gourmand, some would say). My mother was a professional caterer, then a cook, then a cookery teacher. From the age of five I was a regular in her professional kitchen, helping prepare vegetables or stirring a pot. My father's first career was a farmer, then a market gardener. He fished or shot almost every day so my pocket money was earned from the preparation of fish or game for the family table. My father also grew his own fruit and vegetables and so I was weaned on organic produce long before it became modish.

It is no surprise that, since leaving school and home, I have been the cook for fellow flatmates, girlfriends, wife and family – catering, purchasing, preparing ingredients and cooking meals. Cooking for others can be a delight, but the rewards carry with them some major temptations. To cook properly, from scratch using raw ingredients, it is important that everything should be tasted throughout the process. This – and the gourmand in me – has meant that like many of us in the Western world I seem to be forever watching my weight.

Over the years I have fallen for many improbable but tempting diet plans, my bathroom scales fluctuating by as much as 13 kg (28 lb) from any one time to another. Up to a point the diets I followed did work – in the short term. I lost some weight, felt smug when friends and colleagues remarked on my success, and then felt depressed as the weight soon bounced back to where I first started – usually plus some.

Two years ago all this changed.

My wife and I had arranged a four-week holiday in Cape Town, South Africa. This was to be my first visit and I had no real idea of the culinary treats that awaited me. I also had no idea how life changing this visit would become.

South Africa is famous for its seductive and indulgent 'rainbow' cuisine – an eclectic mix of styles and content, inspired by colonisation, immigration and of course, indigenous products. In Cape Town, everybody who can eats out and food is plentiful and inexpensive. A 'bring your own' policy in most restaurants helps sensible diners save even more money on their wine. The combination of large portions and inexpensive wine immediately signalled to me the onset of yet another ballooning waistline. The prospect of a gourmet four-week stay in this beautiful country started to ring alarm bells.

Then I remembered Mount Athos.

Mount Athos in northern Greece is one of the world's most beautiful, unspoilt places and the home to 20 Orthodox monasteries. Shortly before leaving for South Africa I had returned home from a week spent on 'The Holy Mountain' as it is sometimes called. I had been staying as a pilgrim and guest of the monks, living alongside them, walking from monastery to monastery – eating, drinking and, by default, following the monks' diet: the Mount Athos Diet. When I returned home I felt fitter and more relaxed, and looked healthier.

Each monastery is largely self-sufficient, and chiefly as a part of their religious observance and also to preserve food stocks, the monks eat differently on a Monday, Wednesday and Friday. On these three days they eat what we would call a vegan diet: they avoid meat, fish, dairy produce and wine, and they don't use oil to cook. For the remainder of the week they eat dairy, eggs and fish, use olive oil to cook, and drink red wine. One week of living with the Holy Fathers saw me lose 0.9 kg (2 lb) in weight – without trying, and without any lingering sense of deprivation.

Arriving in Cape Town, I took one look at the temptations of the South African diet and thought – no. I have been away for a week, I've lost weight, and I feel much better for it. Instead of chilling out for a month, putting it all back on and returning home bloated, I thought: why not continue following the Mount Athos way of eating vegan for three days of the week?

Everyone thought I was crazy: 'On holiday in a gastronomic heaven like South Africa, and you want to FAST?'

But the monks don't really fast. They eat sensibly and moderately throughout the week, indulging perhaps at the weekend, celebrating one or other of their many Feast Days. So, that is what I did. For four weeks on holiday I avoided meat and dairy produce for three days, and ate sensibly for the remainder of the week. I found it surprisingly easy to incorporate the three vegan days into my week; eating moderately, enjoying dairy products, fish and white meat and wine on the three other days; and feasting on anything I wanted on the final day. To be truthful, any weight loss that I actually achieved while on holiday was counteracted by rather too much beer, and injudicious snacking, but four weeks later I returned home no heavier than when I had left.

I had discovered The Mount Athos Diet.

CHAPTER 1

MOUNT ATHOS – LIFE ON THE HOLY MOUNTAIN

The monks of Mount Athos have been eating the same way for well over 1,000 years. Theirs truly is a 'diet for life'. So, how did this extraordinary place – the Holy Mountain – first begin?

There is evidence that the first Christian hermits settled in Mount Athos in the 7th century. Today, Mount Athos is a self-governing monastic republic, which forms part of the Halkidiki region of Northern Greece, one of three peninsulas that dip south like fingers into the Aegean Sea. A natural ecosystem with rich biodiversity, it is one of the only UNESCO World Heritage sites recognised for both its cultural and natural significance. According to tradition, the Virgin Mary, who after Christ's death had joined the disciples, was sailing with St John the Evangelist towards Cyprus to visit Lazarus. Caught in a sudden storm, their boat was blown on to the Athos peninsula. Mary walked ashore and was immediately overwhelmed by the wild, unspoilt beauty of the mountain. She blessed the land and it became consecrated as the Virgin's Garden and she declared that in future, all female creatures would be barred from Athos. Apart from the wild animals and cats (encouraged in order to keep down the rodent population) Athos has remained a male dominion.

The first Orthodox monastery was founded in AD 866 and today 20 main monasteries remain, plus outlying villages, or *sketes*, and countless individual cells, each occupied by one or two ageing monks. In total, around 2,500 monks live throughout Mount Athos. There is a considerable age range: some monks are well into their nineties, but most are in their thirties and forties. Some have been monks for decades, while others were novices until recently, and all represent a wide cross-section of society. Orthodoxy and nationalism are closely connected: apart from Greek monasteries there are Russian, Serbian and Bulgarian monasteries, which cater largely to their own citizens. Monks themselves come from all over the world, including the USA, Britain, Australia and France.

Despite numerous threats to their existence – rapid technological advances, secularism and political interference – the monks' daily routine and diet have barely changed in the past 1,150 years.

LIFE INSIDE THE MONASTERIES

Monastic life revolves around prayer. Much of the day is spent in the church, conducting services, which can last several hours. Despite having abandoned the world, the chief duty of the monks is to pray for the world although monastic life is not entirely introspective. Several monasteries are closely involved with various outside charitable causes which support refugees, help develop young people, offer drug addicts a new perspective, and raise funds for natural disasters.

The monasteries themselves are surprisingly large and some even appear to resemble small towns. They are walled and gated communities, originally designed to provide protection against marauding pirates and Crusaders who would make every effort to conquer and loot the Holy Mountain of its priceless icons, relics and manuscripts.

Not surprisingly, the daily upkeep of such large and busy communities is laborious. Apart from some help from outside workers, the monks rely on their own talents and are remarkably self-sufficient. Much building restoration and general upkeep is carried out using traditional methods and equipment. Recently, modernity has slowly arrived in the form of 4x4s, telephones and the internet, but Athos remains largely immune from what Henry Adams recognised in the 1890s as 'accelerating change'.

Despite an unavoidable creep towards some features of a 21st-century lifestyle, in most respects the Athos of today remains a world apart. The world of the monasteries still uses the old Julian calendar, meaning that Mount Athos is 13 days behind mainland Greece and the rest of Europe. The monastic liturgical day begins, not at midnight but at sunset, meaning that the monks are five hours ahead of what the monks refer to as 'the World'.

No television, no musical instruments, no advertising hoardings, no news media, no noise, no air pollution. Everything about the monks' world seems aimed at keeping life in the slow lane for as long as is possible. Austere as they may sound to our Western ears these self-imposed anachronisms certainly add to the mystic, other-worldliness of the place and the exclusiveness of the monasteries of Mount Athos forms a core part of their survival.

VISITING THE HOLY MOUNTAIN

Athos is not the easiest place to visit. Firstly, as decreed by the Blessed Virgin Mary, women are barred from entering the Holy Mountain. In addition to Orthodox men who are allowed entry each day, 10 non-Orthodox pilgrims are also granted permission to visit. Visitors apply well ahead for a diamoniterion, an elaborately stamped and signed pass which allows the bearer to stay on Mount Athos for three nights only, in separate monasteries. Reservations for overnight stays in individual monasteries have to be made well in advance, by phone, letter or fax.

Every morning, at 9.45am a ferry departs for Mount Athos, dispensing passengers at various coastal monasteries, which lie on the route to Daphne, a tiny port some two hours down the peninsula. Departing pilgrims are rounded up and the ferry makes its way back to Ouranopoulis, where it first started. This round trip, weather permitting, takes place 365 days of the year.

To maintain this constant flow the monasteries are busy places, catering to the needs of hundreds of visitors throughout the year. No charge is made, or expected, for either accommodation or food. It is the obligation of all monasteries to do their best to take in visiting pilgrims and offer succour and a bed for the night.

MONKS, THEIR GUESTS AND THE DAILY ROUND

The monks' day is divided equally into three: prayer, work and sleep. At the start of each year the Abbot distributes work assignments to all members of the Brotherhood who will retain their allotted job for 12 months, perhaps longer.

There is much to be done. As part of their religion, Orthodox monasteries are obliged to accept pilgrims where they can. The Greek for stranger is *xenios*, which also means 'guest'. Greeting and playing host to strangers was considered important by the early Greeks, who thought that the gods mingled among them, so failing in one's duty as host carried the risk of incurring the wrath of a god disguised as the stranger.

Greeks incorporate *xenia* into their customs and manners and it is now standard practice throughout much (if not all) of Greece. Some monasteries take only a handful of pilgrims; others welcome hundreds per day and these visiting strangers have to be housed and fed. Food needs to be prepared, cooked and served, refectory tables cleared away and re-set for the next meal, facilities need cleaning, beds require a daily linen change.

Many monks rarely leave the confines of their monastery. When they do, it may be to take the ferry to the mainland, or perhaps to visit a neighbouring monastery. Although transport can be found, walking remains the preferred way of getting around the peninsula, which is criss-crossed with ancient, paved Byzantine mule tracks. It can take as much as three to five hours to reach the nearest monastery, double if returning the same day.

The life of a monk might be contemplative and spiritual, but it is also a life kept busy with an endless rota of daily chores: monasticism is never a sedentary occupation. Whatever task has been assigned to a monk, a third of his day is highly active whether on the land, in the kitchens, fishing, restoring buildings, making beds or cleaning.

Tending the gardens, orchards and beehives is also a continuous process. Planting, watering, weeding, training, pruning and harvesting year in, year out is tough for the monks, especially when carried out under an unrelenting Greek sun while clothed from head to foot in black garments. Even so, the monks enjoy gardening, recognising it as one of the best workouts available. Good, old-fashioned aerobic exercise means that it is unusual to see a really chubby monk.

HOW THE MONKS EAT

The Mount Athos Diet is one of the world's best-kept secrets.

Studies have shown that the monasteries of Athos are among the world's healthiest communities. The monks live very long lives, largely free of cancers, cardiovascular disease, diabetes and Alzheimer's. Their way of eating also carries with it an enticing by-product: natural weight loss.

The monks don't count calories, nor do they suffer any of the deprivation commonly associated with the 'fad' diets of the Western world. Theirs is not really a 'diet', more a way of life. They eat good food and drink good wine, and by following age-old principles of using wholesome ingredients, eating in moderation and exercising regularly, they are among the fittest and healthiest people on earth.

Each monastery is largely self-sufficient and very little produce is bought in from the mainland. The monasteries are surrounded by kitchen gardens, orchards, vineyards, beehives and olive groves, and everything produced is organic and seasonal; much time-consuming effort is required to nurture crops and maintain the maximum possible output from the land. Monasteries have their own little harbours, from which to sail their fishing boats. Fishing sorties are usually a prelude to a forthcoming Feast Day, when vast quantities of fish are scaled, gutted and prepared for the pot.

Monastery meals are an extension of the daily religious observance, occurring twice a day – morning and evening. Meals are consumed in silence, as the monks listen to the daily readings from the scriptures (with occasional interruptions from the Abbot). Most meals last around 20 minutes and end when the Abbot rings a bell. Although the monks regard eating as 'refuelling' their food is tasty and varied with soups, greens, beans and pulses, home-produced salads, bread and fruit dominating the menu.

Their pattern of eating remains constant: Mondays, Wednesdays and Fridays are regarded as Fast Days when the diet is essentially vegan – no dairy or animal protein, no wine or olive oil. Fast Day cooking is done with water, rather than oil. Despite some restrictions, a typical Fast Day 'menu' will include plenty of food; it is quite common for food to be left over, to be recycled for the next meal or fed to the monastery cats, nurtured for their rodent-catching skills, so nobody goes hungry.

The remainder of the week (unless there is a Feast Day looming) is given over to Moderation Days when the daily menu expands to include fish, cheese, eggs, yogurt and red wine.

Feast Days are joyous occasions, when home-caught fish dominates the menu, cakes, sweets and even ice cream may be served. These are seen by the monks as 'treats', but even so – always consumed in moderation.

CHAPTER 2

WHAT IS FASTING?

Fasting can take several different forms. If a doctor tells you to fast it means drinking only water and eating nothing at all. In a religious sense, spiritual fasting varies among the different faiths, and the intensity of a fast may depend on how orthodox or devout you are. For example, nothing must pass the lips of Muslims during daylight hours through the month of the Islamic fast of Ramadan, or in the case of Catholicism, no meat should be eaten on Fridays (so fish became the traditional choice).

Fasting doesn't always mean no food. It often means simpler food. In the Greek Orthodox Church this means abstaining from meat, fish or dairy products (cheese, milk, yogurt), and no oil or alcohol. You are eating only what your body needs to function properly and no more. In the case of the Mount Athos Diet, we are following the fasting rules of the monks. For them, fasting means eating in a simple, restrained and modest way, as well as avoiding the excesses of meat, dairy, oil and alcohol. Meals are simple and small, and they don't snack.

To all intents and purposes, the monks are eating a vegan diet on Mondays, Wednesdays and Fridays. But ask any monk why they eat vegan, and they are unlikely to have an answer, primarily because they don't see their diet as being specifically vegan.

The monks do not consider that they have a restricted diet on Fast Days – more a different diet. It is all part of their desire to do things in moderation. Their form of intermittent fasting is a way of giving their bodies a rest, cleansing not only their body, but their mind too. Monks are not particularly interested in the remarkable benefits that fasting can bring: better health, weight control, a longer life. To the monks, these are mildly interesting by-products of a way of life that they have followed for over 1,000 years; monastery food is a means to an end.

Monastery meals are communal affairs, and are always taken in the refectory found opposite the main church doors. This arrangement makes it easy for the monks to incorporate their meals into their liturgical pattern; they are an extension of the church services. Regular fasting offers the monks the chance to subdue any urge to over-indulge, allowing them to concentrate fully on the monk who is charged with reading extracts from the scriptures. Their moderation helps them keep greed at bay: 'Fasting and self-control are virtues'.

FASTING IN THE 21ST CENTURY

Both fasting and the vegan diet have become hugely popular in today's dietary circles, and yet neither is a new concept. As far back as the mid 1800s a Dr Hookey wrote *The No Breakfast Plan*. Veganism was long ago advocated for promoting better health and spiritual development and can be traced back to eastern Mediterranean and ancient Indian societies. The Greek philosopher Pythagoras promoted the vegan way of life over 2,500 years ago while many of the world's religions – Buddhism, Hinduism, Jainism and Shintoism – also advocate vegetarianism and periodic fasting. Periodic fasting has also long been practised by Jews, Christians and Muslims as a form of penance and purification.

Over the past 100 years, medics around the world have cited fasting as a cure for anything from rheumatism to infectious diseases to bowel cleansing.

HOW THE MOUNT ATHOS DIET FAST DAYS CAN CONTRIBUTE TO BETTER HEALTH

There is little doubt that the monks of Mount Athos enjoy long and exceptionally healthy lives, free from many of the ailments that plague the Western world. A relatively slow life enjoyed with a lack of existential cares clearly plays a part in their remarkable health record, but so too does their adherence to three weekly vegan days.

The natural reduction in calories on Fast Days brings with it many health benefits. However, it is our belief that fasting alone does not contribute to the monks' health record. It is the *combination* of fasting and the addition of a further three days of moderation, that helps maintain both physical and mental health.

Fasting (and moderation) let the body rest and cleanse itself. There is an increasing amount of evidence that short periods of fasting can deliver many health benefits. It seems to improve blood pressure (which influences the risk of strokes and heart disease), improve insulin sensitivity (making you less prone to diabetes), improve your blood lipid profile (the fats and cholesterol in your blood), and there is also evidence of it making you live longer, improving brain health and reducing the risk of cancer.

Early evening meals play their part, too. The earlier we eat our final meal of the day, the longer our bodies have time to rest and recuperate. Much of the West seems to regard eating as a 24/7 pastime, whereas the Mount Athos Diet fasting is simply a way of balancing eating differently with eating moderately. It is eminently doable.

The monks of Mount Athos eat this way every week, every month, every year. It is not, for them, a 'diet' in the Western sense; it is a way of life – and its continuity throws up few challenges or a serious risk of 'falling off the wagon'. The yo-yo effects that many modern diet regimes result in simply means that, once the dieter goes back to a 'normal' pattern of eating, body weight comes bouncing back, usually much quicker than it came off.

CHAPTER 3

UNDERSTANDING THE MOUNT ATHOS DIET

WHY IS IT DIFFERENT AND HOW DOES IT WORK?

Studies show that the monks of Mount Athos are among the healthiest people on earth. The Aristotle University of Thessaloniki has conducted research into the health, fitness and longevity of the monks. The findings are startling. Cancers are almost unheard of, especially cancer of the stomach and intestines, the oesophagus and digestive tract, the bladder and prostate. Strokes and cardiac arrests are almost non-existent and Alzheimer's disease is unheard of.

The monks live on average far longer than men on mainland Greece. The monastery graveyards are populated by men who survived well into their eighties or nineties. In two monastery graveyards, researched in May 2013, the average age of the monks buried there was 87 in the first and 89 in the second. The life expectancy of a British male is 79 and a Greek male is 78 (World Health Organisation: 2011).

The monks' unusual longevity is put down to the monastic way of eating which is similar to a typical Greek peasant diet, the so-called Mediterranean diet – a high intake of vegetables, beans and pulses, fruit, nuts, whole grains and olive oil. At the same time, the Mediterranean diet includes a moderate intake of fish, poultry and red wine, and a low intake of dairy products, red meat, processed foods and sweets.

All the food eaten in the monasteries is fresh, organic and seasonal. The monks eat no meat or processed foods, and alternate oil-based meals with water-based meals, giving the stomach a chance to rest three times a week.

The monks of Mount Athos have been eating this way for well over 1,000 years and eating forms part of their religious observance. The Mount Athos Diet has barely changed over the centuries and is here to stay.

WHY YOU WILL LOVE THE MOUNT ATHOS DIET

The Mount Athos Diet is not the usual fixed regime, with strict rules and packets of formula food. It is a sustainable and moderate way of eating. If you already enjoy the delights of fresh, seasonal vegetables and plant-based meals, and savour the clean, light taste of fish and chicken, this diet will suit you well. If on the other hand your shopping list normally includes ready-meals, processed foods, lots of red meat and alcohol, then the Mount Athos Diet promises to be a genuine revelation.

It will only take you two to three weeks to notice how your body and metabolism are responding to subtle changes in your eating and shopping habits. Volunteers who followed the Mount Athos Diet have repeatedly told us that it has brought about a remarkable mind-shift – permanent changes of focus and perception:

- a greater knowledge about and enjoyment of cooking and eating vegetables;

- the lack of hunger pangs;
- the lack of any sense of deprivation;
- less desire for red meat;
- a huge reduction in the consumption of processed foods;
- a flexible eating and dieting schedule;
- a sensible level of alcohol consumption;
- a huge drop in food wastage;
- a significant saving in food and drink bills.

FAD DIETS

Diets come, diets go. It is estimated that in the UK, with 12 million people obese, and a further 24 million overweight, at any one time there are around 27 million people on some form of diet. And many of these diets are what we call 'fad diets'. The term 'fad diet' is faintly scornful, as these diets rapidly become popular then, just as rapidly, fall out of fashion. Remember the Grapefruit Diet? The Cabbage Soup Diet? The Blood Type Diet? The Zone Diet? The Atkins Diet? The Dukan Diet? The South Beach Diet? All hugely successful in their day – in the short term. 'Fad' often also means a diet that is not based on the generally accepted principles of healthy eating, and is often found to be largely unworkable or impossible to keep to.

THE DEPRIVATION TRAP

Most diets ultimately fail because they are centred on deprivation in some form. Most people are capable of changing their shopping habits and eating patterns for a short while. An initial, intoxicating euphoria greets the onset of any new diet, then something gets in the way. If it's not good old-fashioned temptation – that irresistible urge to open the refrigerator door every time you walk past, or to check the biscuit tin for any last remaining occupants – then it's social pressure. Major difficulties can arise when confronted by a limited restaurant menu, or a plate of food put before you by well-meaning friends in their home, not to mention the nibbles table at a party, so tempting to graze from throughout the evening.

Deprivation simply heightens the urge to have whatever it is that you are missing. The very fact that the latest diet bans you from having something you love soon makes it become the focus of your attention. If deprived long enough, temptation becomes unbearable and 'just a little bit won't do me any harm' quickly slides into a full-blown binge. No chocolate for a week – then two whole bars in one go. After this, and having defaulted a few more times, most dieters end up thinking: 'The hell with it. This diet isn't working. I give up.'

It's not the diets that are at fault; it's the unnatural and continuous bouts of deprivation they make you endure. The reason crash or fad diets usually fail is that they involve savage cutbacks in calorie intake and serious deprivation, forcing the body to break down muscle to use as energy. Crash diets inevitably result in an apparent loss of weight, but very often, this weight loss is due to a reduction in glycogen and protein, as well as fat. Eventually, the body strives to preserve the depleted energy stores and the initial weight loss starts to plateau. The lower your muscle mass, the lower your metabolism, making it far easier to put body fat back on when coming off the diet. Diets such as this always work for a short while but ultimately your body thinks it's starving and seeks every opportunity to regain the weight lost. Yo-yo dieting is a metabolic roller coaster.

If that isn't enough to put you off, apart from providing a quick fix through poor nutrition the rapid weight loss resulting from a crash diet also results in a loss of supportive fat beneath the skin, which, in turn, can lead to wrinkles.

THE REMARKABLE EFFECTS OF ABSTINENCE

The Mount Athos Diet is not about depriving yourself over long periods. It is not a denial diet. No calorie counting here: monks don't count calories – the only things they count are the knots on their prayer ropes. Follow the diet for a few weeks and quite rapidly your whole attitude to eating will change. Severe hunger pangs and consequent binge eating will become a thing of the past. Your view of highly processed supermarket lasagne will change forever. Food wastage will be cut to a minimum, as there is little or no uneaten food left over to get thrown away. The Mount Athos Diet will put you firmly back in charge of your life and promises you little or no sense of guilt or lingering deprivation.

The underlying reason why the Mount Athos Diet will help make sure you don't pile on the pounds after you have reached your target weight is that within a matter of two to three weeks it leads you automatically to reassess what you eat. It is not so much a diet as a step change in the way we think about food and how we consume it. How it shapes our lives and fine-tunes our health. It is born out of a perfect storm of factors: it is enjoyable, flexible and, above all, doable.

For the monks, food is all about creation, not convenience. No ready-meals or processed foods ever enter a monastery. The monks take time in their kitchens to produce tasty and nourishing meals, using seasonal organic ingredients and herbs mostly grown in their own fields, orchards and olive groves. The monks grow their own wheat and make their own daily whole-grain bread.

Nor are the monks teetotal. Over half their meals are accompanied by their home-produced red wine, decanted from huge storage vats into bottles for the table.

The monks of Mount Athos don't do diets. What we call in this book 'The Mount Athos Diet' is simply a way of eating which has sustained the Greek Orthodox monks for well over 1,000 years. It has kept them slim, fit and unusually healthy throughout their long lives. As you start to enjoy the flexibility and lack of deprivation, which the Mount Athos Diet promises, weight loss accompanied by a raised activity level, and ultimately better health, will follow naturally.

WINDING BACK THE CLOCK FOR A SLIMMER, HEALTHIER, LONGER LIFE

The Mount Athos Diet is that of our great-grandparents. Think back to the 19th and early 20th centuries. At that time processed food did not exist. Ingredients were bought from local specialist shops; there was no such thing as a take-away or a 'ready-meal'; burger joints and pizza parlours had yet to be invented; vegetables and fruit were strictly seasonal; chemical colourants and preservatives non-existent; highly toxic synthetic pesticides, herbicides and fungicides were virtually unknown.

Our forebears ate a diet rich in vegetables and fruit, pulses and beans, all of which we, in the 21st century, frequently regard as 'superfoods'. Portion sizes were modest. Meat was expensive and regarded as a treat and, when eaten, was supplemented by copious amounts of seasonal vegetables. Food items that were really cheap were also very good for the Victorians. Root vegetables, onions, watercress, beetroot and cabbage were both plentiful and organic. Inexpensive oily fish and seafood were high on the menu and pulses and nuts were favourite ingredients. In the Western world of today we have allowed ourselves to become overfed and undernourished.

One of Britain's favourite supermarkets sells a beef lasagne containing no fewer than 32 ingredients. (The lasagne recipe in *The Silver Spoon*, Italy's cookery 'bible', has 11 ingredients.) What would granny have made of this phenomenon?

THE MOUNT ATHOS DIET IN SUMMARY

The Mount Athos Diet is a Western modification of the way the monks eat. The monks have self-imposed, limited resources; they work from a different calendar; their 'time zone' is five hours adrift from what the monks call 'the World'. Those of us who dwell outside the 'Holy Mountain' enjoy the benefits of a completely different world, one that offers a far wider range of foodstuffs, ingredients and sources from which to acquire them. The monks' eating patterns are entwined with their religious practices and offer little or no flexibility. We Westerners generally eat three meals a day, often at different times. For the diet to work for ourselves we must accept that it is impractical to follow the monks' way of life and eating patterns to the letter.

The fasting pattern that the monks follow is the core principle of the Mount Athos Diet. When following the diet you 'fast' on three alternate days a week, you eat 'moderately' on three other days, and on one day of the week you can 'feast', eating and drinking what you like. The Fast Days are low-fat vegan – so you don't eat meat, fish, chicken or dairy products and keep oil to an absolute minimum. No alcohol can be drunk on Fast Days and you need to keep your portions small. Overall the diet promotes lots of fruit and vegetables, eating more beans, lentils, nuts and seeds, and keeping the empty calories in fatty, sugary foods to a minimum.

WHAT DO WE MEAN BY MODERATION?

Monks are not in a position to eat or drink immoderately. They have neither the resources nor the time. It is this adherence to a moderate diet which contributes hugely to their lack of disease, their weight management and their long lives.

The monks' lifestyle calls for them to eat only twice a day; they don't have seconds, they don't snack and they rarely eat sweet things. However, in our world the monks' regime is impractical for those of us who have busy schedules dictated by family and work requirements. Our breakfasts are often taken at speed or skipped altogether, we eat on the go, we snack at the desk and as a result often compensate by eating and drinking immoderately in the evening.

Start your day with a good breakfast, which will help you to avoid snacking or overindulging for the rest of the day. Above all – watch those portion sizes.

MAXIMUM FLEXIBILITY IS ALWAYS YOUR CHOICE

Most diets are strict to the point of being inflexible. Not so on the Mount Athos Diet. As long as you incorporate three Fast Days and three Moderation Days within your week, all will be fine and no guilt need ensue.

The monks fast on intermittent days, but this may not be practical for your situation. Move your Fast Days around to suit your working and social life. For instance, your personal variation of the Mount Athos Diet plan may incorporate Monday, Wednesday and Thursday as your Fast Days and Sunday as your Feast Day. Ideally, don't have more than two Fast Days together, but the choice is always yours.

IS THE MOUNT ATHOS DIET FOR YOU?

Ask yourself these questions. If the answer to most of the questions is 'yes' then the Mount Athos Diet is certainly the one for you.

Do you want to:

- Lose weight steadily and safely?
- Stay slim for the rest of your life?
- Say goodbye to deprivation?
- Avoid for evermore calorie counting?
- Eat and live a healthier life?
- Reduce your risk of disease?
- Feel and look younger?
- Save money on food and drink?
- Enjoy a truly flexible diet?
- Change your approach to food forever?

Sticking to a diet is usually hard work, but not the Mount Athos Diet. It is an entirely natural way of eating which results in steady weight loss and can make you change your eating habits forever.

CHAPTER 4

THE BENEFITS OF THE MOUNT ATHOS DIET

The health of the monks and the food they eat inspired this book. While it is impossible to make absolute health claims about any diet, the Mount Athos Diet will help you lose weight and improve your health with advice that's in line with current recommendations and knowledge about eating well for your body and for the planet.

A MEDITERRANEAN DIET FOR GOOD HEALTH AND A LONG LIFE

The research study that first uncovered the benefits of the Mediterranean diet over the American and North European diets was the Seven Countries Study. This major longitudinal study started over 50 years ago by Ancel Keys and colleagues who examined the health outcomes of more than 13,000 middle-aged men. They learnt that men from the Greek island of Crete had lower rates of cardiovascular disease than those in other countries.

Since this study, not only has the Mediterranean diet been shown in multiple research studies to improve hypertension, heart disease and stroke risk, the diet may lower the risk of diabetes, various types of cancer, obesity and even reduce cognitive decline, dementia and Alzheimer's. Some studies have even found that elderly people who switched to a Mediterranean diet on average lived longer than those who didn't. It seems that not only is a Mediterranean diet beneficial to people *with* cardiovascular disease and hypertension, it also helps to *prevent it* in those with no signs of disease.

The traditional 'Mediterranean diet' refers to the way people ate in the parts of the Mediterranean studied by Keys in the early 1960s, including Crete, other parts of Greece, Spain and southern Italy. The diet is high in fruits, vegetables, cereals, potatoes, poultry, beans, nuts, fish, dairy products, small quantities of red meat (only four to five times a month), moderate alcohol consumption (drunk with meals) and olive oil. In Greece intake of milk is relatively low but the consumption of cheese and yogurt is high. Feta cheese is added regularly to salads and to accompany vegetable stews.

In many of the places included in the Seven Countries Study, diets have started to 'modernise', including more processed foods and drinks with added fats, sugars and salt. However, the monks living on Mount Athos, whose diets haven't changed for hundreds of years, still eat in the simple traditional way.

AVOIDING SUGAR

Up until now the focus of healthy eating advice has very much been on fat, particularly saturated fat, with sugar almost as an afterthought. Its only fault was deemed to be that it was 'empty calories', so not the wisest place to get calories from. The logic is that as we become less active we need fewer calories, therefore you should get those calories from foods with lots of nutrients in them, not sugar. The other problem with sugar was that it decayed your teeth.

There is a growing consensus that sugar actually plays a wider role in our poor health. Eating too much sugar seems to affect your metabolism, as well as your waistline, leading to metabolic syndrome, which results in conditions like obesity, diabetes and heart disease. In the book *Fat Chance: The bitter truth about sugar* endocrinologist Dr Robert Lustig extensively explains the science behind the problem. He highlights the addictive nature of sugar, and as you may have noticed yourself, the more sugar you eat, the more you need of it to taste sweetness.

Sticking to sugar and sweet treats only on your Feast Days will help you lose weight and improve your health.

ALCOHOL

The Mount Athos Diet will help you to bring your alcohol intake to levels that are potentially positive for your health rather than detrimental. Alcohol may be significantly contributing to your excessive calorie intake and weight gain, so limiting the amount of the 'empty calories' you drink can make a real impact.

If you currently exceed the recommended limits of not regularly drinking more than 2–3 units per day for women and 3–4 units per day – and this isn't much compared to many people's intake – and if you drink almost every day of the week, the diet will help you reduce this and break bad habits. Like snacking, you need to change the rut of your routine that can lead you to drink too much. (See Chapter 12 for a full explanation of alcohol units.)

Following the Mount Athos Diet will help you to regulate your drinking to a level that may actually be beneficial to your health – especially your heart. As the monks do, the diet includes moderate amounts (2 units) of red wine on three days of the week, and research suggests that alcohol at these levels may offer heart health benefits. Remember the 'moderation' point though and don't overdo it.

CANCER PREVENTION

About a third of the most common cancers could be prevented through eating a healthy diet, being physically active and maintaining a healthy weight. The World Cancer Research Fund (WCRF) continually reviews all the evidence relating to cancer and its prevention and have summarised it in 10 key recommendations. Five of them relate to food and all of them are principles of the Mount Athos Diet.

WCRF food recommendations to reduce your risk of cancer:

- **energy density:** avoid sugary drinks. Limit consumption of energy dense foods (particularly processed foods high in added sugar, or low in fibre, or high in fat);
- **plant foods**: eat more of a variety of vegetables, fruits, whole grains, and pulses, such as beans;
- **meat:** limit consumption of red meats (such as beef, pork and lamb) and avoid processed meats;
- **alcohol:** if consumed at all, limit alcoholic drinks to two for men and one for women a day;
- **salt:** limit consumption of salty foods and foods processed with salt (sodium).

LESS MEAT IS GOOD FOR THE ENVIRONMENT

When you follow the Mount Athos Diet you will be eating fewer animal products, and reducing your impact on the world's resources (unless you are a vegan already). World-wide, nearly 42 kg (93 lb) of meat is produced per person every year, and it's now widely acknowledged that this is putting a significant strain on the environment. In the UK we eat, on average, just under 80 kg (176 lb) meat per person per year while in the US, people consume 125 kg (276 lb). In Greece today people eat the same amount of meat as in the UK, but in the 1960s when the Seven Countries Study started, the average person ate just 22 kg (49 lb) per year.

Compared to growing crops, rearing animals for food results in a lot more greenhouse gas emissions, water use and land requirements. So by following the Mount Athos Diet and reducing the amount of meat and dairy you eat, you will dramatically reduce the impact of what you eat on the environment. Plant-based foods are a better choice when considering any ethical or environmental aspect of nutrition.

Eating the amount of meat we do in the world today, it just wouldn't be possible for everyone to switch to organic and free-range, as there wouldn't be room in the world to rear the animals. The industrial livestock systems needed to meet our demands are not a long-term viable option; as well as the concerns about the welfare conditions the animals have to endure, these farms require the use of large amounts of land to feed the animals, which threatens global food security. Plus there are many more problems with this type of farming, such as antibiotic resistance, water pollution and soil erosion.

The livestock sector accounts for 18 per cent of the world's carbon emissions, and with the additional concerns about global food security, it's no surprise that we keep hearing our politicians, the UN and environmentalists calling for a reduction in the amount of meat we consume – even if it is just one meat-free day a week.

A comparison of the carbon dioxide (CO_2) produced when producing 1 kg (2¼ lb) of beef compared to 1 kg (2¼ lb) of tofu is dramatic. A Dutch study found that 1 kg (2¼ lb) of beef (Dutch) produces 22 kg (49 lb) CO_2, while the same amount of beef reared in Brazil produces 335 kg (739 lb) CO_2 (which is equivalent to driving an average car for more than 1,600 km/994 miles). On the other hand, protein-rich tofu, which is made from soya beans, produces just 4 kg (9 lb) CO_2.

Eating less meat and moving to a more plant-based diet will free up agricultural land for growing trees and other vegetation, which will absorb carbon dioxide from the atmosphere, as well as producing more crops for people. Currently over a third of all cereal crops and over 90 per cent of the entire soya grown in the world is used for animal feed.

Oxfam has reviewed the impact that meat production has on the world's fragile water supplies. They have calculated the amount of water needed to produce beef and beans to illustrate the differing impact. It takes a staggering 6,810 litres (1,497 gallons) of water to produce 500 g (1 lb 2 oz) of beef. Whereas growing 500 g (1 lb 2 oz) of beans only takes 818 litres (179 gallons) of water. So by swapping beef for beans in one family meal you are saving nearly 6,000 litres (1,319 gallons) of water (that's more than 17 bathtubs filled with water).

BETTER FOR YOU, BETTER FOR THE PLANET

Various scientists are of the opinion that eating a less processed, more natural, home-cooked diet will improve health and reduce your risk of the chronic diseases of the West – heart disease, stroke, diabetes and cancer.

It's hard to argue with the Mount Athos approach to eating. It makes sense for your health and for the environment in many different ways. And if you follow it as laid out in this book, it can help you lose weight in a regular, sensible and relatively easy way, teaching you habits and a way of cooking that can help you keep your weight in check for the rest of your life.

CHAPTER 5

THE MOUNT ATHOS DIET PLAN

The Mount Athos Diet is not about counting calories or unhealthy extremes, it is centred on changing your approach to food. As well as helping you to lose and maintain your weight, this diet is very likely to be cheaper, healthier and better for the planet than what you were eating before.

The diet should also help you ditch the 'diet' mentality, and value and respect the food you eat. With a weekly Feast Day, you don't have to say 'no' for weeks on end. You will instead develop a more balanced approach to food, thinking 'not today', rather than 'never'.

The diet is a modified version of the way the monks eat on Mount Athos and reflects the greater range of ingredients available to us in the UK. We offer a wider range of recipes, inspired by cuisines from around the world that have full-flavoured dishes using little or no animal protein, such as Asian and Middle Eastern, as well as Mediterranean.

When you start building the diet into your daily life, think about the monks, their monastic eating habits and the active way they live their lives. Their religion and circumstances on Mount Athos result in a very modest diet that is grown and sourced around them, with a variation of Fast Days, Moderation Days and occasional Feast Days.

THE THREE EATING PATTERNS

The varying pattern of diet days is the core principle of the Mount Athos Diet. There are three different types of days – Fast Days, Moderation Days and Feast Days.

FAST DAYS
(three days a week, for example Monday, Wednesday and Friday)
- No animal protein, i.e. dairy, eggs, red meat, fish or chicken.
- No alcohol.
- Oil and cooking fats kept to a minimum.

Can eat: unlimited vegetables and fruit, also beans, lentils, pulses, tofu, nuts and seeds. Limited portions of pasta, wholegrain bread, potatoes and rice.

MODERATION DAYS
(three days a week, for example Tuesday, Thursday and Sunday)
Everything you eat on Fast Days, plus:

- dairy products, eggs, fish and chicken (but no red meat);
- olive oil;
- alcohol: 2 units of (preferably) red wine a day.

FEAST DAY
(one day a week, for example Saturday)
On this day you can eat and drink what you like. This is your chance to eat meat and indulge a little. However, it is likely

that what you choose to eat on Feast Days will change, the longer you follow the diet.

MOUNT ATHOS DIET PRINCIPLES

The pattern of intermittent fasting days and one Feast Day a week, as described above, is central to the Mount Athos Diet. However, additional dietary principles, taken from the monks' way of life, have guided the diet and are a healthy and conscientious way to live and eat.

- Keep salt and processed foods to a minimum.
- Keep butter and cream to a minimum.
- Keep sugar and sugary drinks to a minimum and preferably avoid altogether.
- Cut down on fruit juice and substitute with water.
- Snack only on fruit, vegetables, nuts and dry crackers.
- Eat organically produced food when you have a choice.
- Grow your own vegetables if possible.
- Buy your meat and fish from reliable, traceable sources.
- Exercise regularly (for example, a brisk walk of 30–40 minutes a day will help keep your weight down).
- Drink plenty of water.
- Be flexible when you need to be. Move Fast Days around to fit in with changing social plans.

OVERVIEW

Following the Mount Athos Diet is about learning a new way of eating. Your health will benefit from eating lots of fruits and vegetables, beans, grains and nuts. Combining this with the low amount of meat, limited dairy, the inclusion of fish, and the use of olive oil as the main fat in your diet, your nutrient balance will be rich in monounsaturated and polyunsaturated fats, and rich in the known and unknown protective elements that a plant-based diet offers (including fibre, vitamins, minerals and phytochemicals).

It is also as much about what you don't eat as what you do. Avoiding processed foods, snacks and drinks will help you to eat less of the fat, salt and sugar that goes into many of them. By eating less processed foods, we hope the result is that you cook more for yourself, creating wholesome meals made from fresh ingredients. This way you will get maximum nutrition from the food (and calories) you eat.

Most people can only eat a limited amount of fat and sugar before the additional calories will influence their weight. Therefore it makes sense to use your fat and sugar calories to increase the palatability of nutrient-dense foods rather than to consume foods or drinks that are mainly just fat or sugar. For example, it's better to consume fat in the form of courgettes sautéed in olive oil and garlic, rather than a packet of crisps. Or it is better to sprinkle a teaspoon of sugar on some fruit rather than have a few sips of cola (one can contains 8 teaspoons of sugar).

THE DIET DAYS IN DETAIL

FAST DAYS

For three days a week you need to fast in the way the Mount Athos monks do. The monks adhere to the strict rules of Greek Orthodox fasting when no meat, eggs, dairy products, fish or oil should be consumed, as well as no alcohol. In addition to choosing from a limited range of foods, you also need to eat as little as possible – think restrained, small portions that are much smaller than what you normally eat.

On Fast Days you are essentially following a low-fat, teetotal, vegan diet. So just like vegans, it's good to learn to love vegetable sources of protein, such as lentils and beans like chickpeas, butter beans and kidney beans, tofu, nuts and seeds. Our collection of Fast Day recipes (see pages 133–186) will help you to create simple, tasty meals with these ingredients. As the principles of Fast Days are low-fat vegan, you can also search for more recipes that meet this criterion, expanding the range of recipes you can cook even further online or in other cookbooks. However, don't be tempted to go down the fake 'alternatives' route, such as vegan cheese or vegan yogurt. These often contain a lot of added fat and/or sugar, and are highly processed. It's better and more in the spirit of the diet to stick to simple vegan recipes.

You will be eating small amounts of a restricted range of foods on Fast Days, but the good news is that it's only for three days a week. So just work out the best pattern that suits you and be as strict with yourself as possible. Expect to feel a bit hungry when you go to bed … it's a good sign.

The Food Rules For Fast Days
Unlimited
When you are fasting you should always be careful about the amount of food you are eating, trying to limit it as much as possible. However, the following are unlimited:

- vegetables (except avocados and potatoes) – pack your meals with as much as you can

- fruit
- herbal/fruit teas
- water
- spices, herbs and pepper – use these to create tasty meals on fasting days

In Moderation

Fasting meals can contain all the following, but still remember that you should be eating small amounts. No meal should be more than what you can cup in your two hands.

Carbohydrates aren't out of bounds. It's fine to eat carbs on your fasting days, but limit the amount and opt for whole grains where possible. The main way to keep a check on yourself is to compare it to what you usually eat – it should be less, as little as you can.

Moderation foods are:

- potatoes
- pasta
- grains – rice, bulgur wheat, couscous, quinoa, barley, oats
- bread – preferably wholemeal
- plain crackers, oat cakes, breadsticks
- fruit juice (limit to no more than 2 small glasses per day)
- avocados (no more than half per day)
- pulses – peas, lentils, beans, such as chickpeas, butter beans, kidney beans (small portions)
- olives and olive oil spray (use sparingly)
- honey (use sparingly)

- condiments and sauces – such as Thai chilli sauce or tomato ketchup (use sparingly)
- dried fruits, nuts and seeds (no more than a handful a day)
- tea and coffee – without milk and sugar
- salt – limit this as much as you can

NOT Allowed

On fasting days your diet will be limited. If you look through this list and get worried that you won't know what to eat and what to cook on these days – see our Fasting Recipes (pages 133–186) and Menu Planner sections (pages 255–243) for lots of tips and ideas.

Don't eat:

- dairy – milk, cheese, butter, yogurt, cream, fromage frais
- meat – beef, pork, all meat products (burgers, sausages, bacon, ham, etc.)
- fish and shellfish – including prawns, squid, fish products (like fish fingers)
- eggs
- chips, fried foods, pastry, pies
- crisps and other snack foods
- biscuits, cakes, pastries, croissants, flapjacks, etc.
- sweets, chocolate and confectionery
- sugar and sugary drinks (such as cola, lemonade, energy drinks)
- alcohol – wine, beer, cider, spirits, cocktails
- oils and fats (including coconut cream and coconut milk)
- mayonnaise and fatty salad dressings

MODERATION DAYS

What you can eat on these days is more varied than on Fast Days, but ensure it's all in moderation, and keep your portions small. In addition to what is allowed on Fast Days, you can have dairy products, eggs, fish and chicken (but not red meat). Fats and oils are allowed, but preferably use olive oil and keep quantities limited. You can have 2 units of alcohol (preferably red wine). This doesn't mean two large glasses of red wine (see Chapter 12 on Alcohol to find out more about units).

The Food Rules For Moderation Days
Unlimited

As on every day of the Mount Athos Diet, the following foods can be eaten in unlimited amounts:

- fruit
- vegetables (except avocados and potatoes)
- herbal/fruit teas
- water
- spices, herbs and pepper

In Moderation

On Moderation Days the range of foods you can eat is broader and more varied, but red meat and meat products are still avoided, as well as fatty and sugary foods and drinks. As the monks do, you can enjoy a glass of red wine with one of your meals.

You can eat:

- grains – rice, bulgur wheat, couscous, barley, oats, quinoa
- pulses – beans and lentils
- nuts and seeds

- bread – preferably wholemeal
- crackers, oatcakes, breadsticks
- pasta
- potatoes
- avocados
- fruit juices
- olives
- honey
- Greek yogurt (or natural yogurt)
- semi-skimmed and skimmed milk
- cheese (a piece no bigger than a matchbox)
- small amount of butter
- eggs
- seafood
- chicken
- olive oil
- alcohol – preferably red wine (2 units per day – which is equivalent to a 175 ml (6 fl oz) standard glass of red wine), drunk with a meal
- dried fruits and nuts
- salt – limit this as much as you can

Not Allowed

- red meat and meat products (such as sausages, burgers, ham, bacon, pâté)
- chips, fried foods, pastry, pies
- sugar and sugary drinks (and it's better to drink water rather than diet drinks)
- crisps and other snack foods
- sweets and confectionery
- cakes, biscuits, croissants, pastries

FEAST DAYS

One day of the week you can have a break from your strict and limited way of eating, and you can 'feast' – indulging in whatever you fancy. Save these days for when you eat out, celebrate with friends or want to do some baking, for example.

The beauty of the Mount Athos Diet is that you don't need to say no to everything and everyone all the time, and you don't have to endure a long-term feeling of deprivation, which is hard to stick with. You can actually enjoy a party or a piece of cake without feeling guilty about what you are doing, because you know that you will be back on to a Fast Day very soon. Feast Days help to limit the problems of deprivation and guilt common in other diets.

When developing this diet we have also been interested to see how people's preferences change over time. While you may expect to go completely over the top on a Feast Day, you will probably find that what you want to eat and drink on these days slowly changes, and you will be craving less sweet and fatty foods over time. That's a very positive effect of the diet as well.

WILL I BE MISSING ANY NUTRIENTS IF I FOLLOW THE DIET?

Protein: most people eat more protein than their body needs. Although you are probably going to be cutting back on meat, you will be eating more vegetarian sources of protein, such as beans, lentils, nuts, seeds or tofu, in addition to a certain amount of fish, chicken and cheese.

Calcium: dairy products are the main source of calcium in the average UK diet. Dark, leafy greens are a good alternative source, such as pak choi, kale and broccoli, as well as almonds.

Iron: red meat is a good source of iron that is easy to absorb. When eating vegetarian sources of iron, for example beans, lentils and dark leafy greens, it's best to consume foods containing vitamin C at the same time, as this increases the absorption of this different form of iron dramatically. So for example, have a small glass of fruit juice with a meal, or the vitamin C may come from the vegetables or salad you serve with a meal.

If you are concerned that your diet is deficient in any nutrients and you want to take a supplement, it is best to stick to a generic multivitamin and mineral supplement, with nutrients at or around 100 per cent RDA levels, not in mega doses.

CHAPTER 6

SET YOUR SIGHTS ON SUCCESS

HOW TO PROGRAMME YOUR BRAIN AND PHYSIOLOGY TO LOSE WEIGHT AND STAY HEALTHY

You are moulding your tomorrow based on what you do today. You can determine what your future holds based on how much time and energy you spend working on yourself now. Find out what it is you want, and go after it as if your life depends on it. Why? Because it does.

Les Brown, author and motivational speaker

You can choose to stay as you are or decide to become what you are capable of becoming. But how to be a successful dieter when surrounded by temptations – and by people who are not on your diet? The answer is both simple and challenging – you set yourself realistic goals and stick to them. That's the easy part. We will address the challenging bit a little later.

Most people agree that objective setting is important but do little or nothing about it. A recent study in the *Journal of the American Dietetic Association* reported that good goal setting increases your chances of reaching your diet objective by 84 per cent.

Setting objectives for ourselves is seldom easy. For an objective to be achieved we have to work at it; it means continued effort, commitment and self-discipline. We have to know our weaknesses and recognise and deal with the many barriers that will block our path to success, but barriers can be a good thing, as they also represent a test of your resolve. Brick walls are there for a reason. They let you prove how badly you want things.

FIVE GOOD REASONS FOR SETTING YOURSELF MOUNT ATHOS DIET GOALS

- They will help ensure your success. Successful people around the world share a common characteristic: they believe in goal setting.
- People with clear goals succeed because they know where they are going.
- Goal setting is arguably the single most important aspect of the dieting process.
- Setting clearly defined, well-formed goals actually works.
- People who commit to written goals for themselves are demonstrably more successful as a result.

SO – WHAT DO YOU WANT TO ACHIEVE?

Before you commence your plan to follow the Mount Athos Diet, think clearly about your objectives. What do you want to happen – the end result of losing weight, feeling younger, living longer? Here are some questions that you may want to ask yourself even before you start to formulate and write down your well-formed outcome statement.

Which is most important to me?

- Weight loss?
- Feeling younger?
- Living longer?
- Eating better?
- Drinking less alcohol?
- Improving my health and vigour?
- Reducing the chances of chronic disease?
- Maintaining a healthy body weight?
- Being able to get back into much-loved clothing?
- Saving money on food and drink bills?
- Feeling more confident and attractive in social situations?

THE FOUR STEPS TO SUCCESS – SETTING YOURSELF CONSCIOUS OBJECTIVES

Step one – think positively

Start by eradicating all those limiting beliefs: it'll never work; I've tried this before; I'm too old, etc.

Make certain that your objective is stated in the positive; think of what you want rather than what you don't want.

Example: 'I don't want to look like this any longer.'
Q. 'How would you prefer to look?'
A. 'I want to look thinner and younger.'

You can see that 'I don't want to look like this any longer' gives you nothing specific to go towards, but 'looking thinner and younger' are measureable goals.

Step two – put yourself in charge

Do you own the objective or is it another person's? For example, if your partner tells you 'I think you should lose weight' that is their objective, not yours. Think of the part you will play in achieving the outcome. Make certain that the possibility of achievement is within your control, not someone else's.

Step three – be very specific about the ways in which you will ensure your objective is met

State your objective in manageable proportions that also make it seem real: something definite to go for, which begins to suggest genuine actions towards getting to the outcome.

Think of your short-term goals, your medium-term goals and your long-term goals, for example:

- Short-term: To lose 11 kg (25 lb) in three months.
- Medium-term: To devise a sensible exercise plan for myself.
- Long-term: To maintain my eventual weight loss.

Step four – what evidence will prove to you that you have achieved your objective?

What sensory evidence will you experience – the information that your senses will tell you when you have got what you want. This will make your objective far more real and compelling.

Use these senses:

- sight – the evidence you will see (a slimmer reflection in your mirror?);
- sound – the evidence you will hear ('Wow! You've lost weight. How did you do it?');

- feeling (1) – the evidence you will sense emotionally (a sustained glow of satisfaction?);
- feeling (2) – the evidence you will touch (your toes?).

There are, of course, five senses and you may be able to include taste and smell in your evidence check. Recently, I was helping a friend, Amy, to set some dieting objectives. She wanted to lose sufficient weight to take up the offer of a holiday of a lifetime to Greece. Until now, she had been so ashamed of her body image that there was no chance of her parading on a beach in front of tanned and toned twenty-somethings. When it came to deciding what evidence would prove to her that she had achieved her weight-loss objective I asked her:

Question. 'What will you see, hear and feel both inside and outside that will let you know that you have achieved your objective?'

Answer. 'I will see the cloudless blue sky above me and hear the soft sound of waves. Greek music is wafting through the olive grove and I hear the clink of ice in the glass in my hand. I will feel the sun on my body and the weight of the cold glass in my hand. I will smell sun oil and taste the wine in the glass.'

Wow. Amy had formed a very clear, sensory concept of where her diet was taking her. Her answer was way more substantial and robust than 'I'll know when I am successful', which usually means just the opposite. (Later that summer Amy called me. 'That goal-setting exercise we did together was amazing. As soon as I got to the island and lay on the beach it all came flooding back to me. The sights and sounds, the smells and tastes – were all just as I had visualised. It made the hairs on the back of my neck stand up. Magic!')

MOUNT ATHOS DIET OBJECTIVES – THE FOUR-STEP PATH SUMMARISED

1 Write down your goals. Check to make sure they are stated positively.
2 Make sure you have full control over the outcome.
3 Be specific about the ways you will go about achieving your objective.
4 Ask yourself: what evidence will I see, hear, feel, smell or taste which will confirm that I have achieved my objective?

WHY CREATIVE VISUALISATION WORKS

Your creative imagination is capable of producing a physical response. In his book *Psycho-Cybernetics; a new way to get more living out of life*, Dr Maxwell Maltz clarified a profound truth: the subconscious mind does not know the difference between a real and an imagined event. In other words, it is perfectly possible to programme our brains towards achieving a set goal. A good example of this phenomenon is sport. For instance, before taking a shot top golfers mentally 'watch' the ball going into the hole then track the successful shot backwards, to where they are positioned in order to understand what they have to do to get the ball in the hole.

If all this sounds like a load of West Coast American mumbo jumbo try this little experiment. Close your eyes and relax.

Imagine that you are holding a fat, ripe lemon. Weigh it in your hand, feel its coolness, savour the strong citrus smell given off from its waxy skin. Now, imagine that you are cutting into it with a sharp knife. Peel away the skin and notice the juice already seeping out from the glistening segments. Feel your mouth salivating as you imagine biting into a piece, the juices squirting out on to your tongue. Your creative imagination alone has induced a physical response; your mouth starts to produce saliva.

Maxwell Maltz said that one of the great truths in the world of humans is that you become what you think about all day long. If you see yourself bright, cheerful and successful, it will work wonders in your life. If you see yourself pessimistically as a failure and unsuccessful, you have created a blueprint for your subconscious mind to follow. And if you see yourself as a successful dieter ... a slim person ... a healthier, younger-looking you ...

Not only does your subconscious mind not know the difference between a real and an imagined event, it does not choose between what's good for you or what's bad for you. It just follows the orders you give it – 'I'll have a doughnut, and then two more' – just like a computer follows the programming that goes in. If you put rubbish in, you get rubbish out. It's as true for our bodies as it is for our computers.

USE YOUR 'INNER VOICE' TO KEEP ON TRACK

It is quite common, and normal, to hear voices in our heads. Sometimes the voice may be encouraging: Go on, you know you can do it. Or admonishing: You know you shouldn't ...

the voice we hear regulates our behaviour and can play an important role in motivating us.

Athletes conventionally give themselves pep talks. Tennis player Andy Murray credits a pep talk for his US Open victory in 2012. Playing against his friend (and sometime nemesis) Novak Djokovic, Murray appeared on course for yet another humiliating heartbreak after squandering a two-set lead.

'It had got to me,' Murray recalled, 'I had played four grand slam finals before playing Novak in New York and had only won one set. Wherever I walked, I walked with hunched shoulders and with my head down.

'I think in my own mind I had bought the idea that I was not a real winner until I had won a grand slam. I was very negative in my own mind at the end of the fourth set at the US Open. My self-belief was pretty low.'

Then Murray took a toilet break from the match, thinking to himself: 'Why do I keep losing these finals? Do I lack something? How on earth did I squander a two-set lead?'

'So I started talking to myself. "You are not losing this match," I said to myself. "You are not losing this match. You are not going to let this one slip. This is your time."'

Murray then felt something change inside him. He knew he could win. He marched back on court and had no trouble closing out the final set 6–2. Our inner voice is a powerful tool of self-regulation and motivation.

DEALING WITH NEGATIVE THOUGHTS

Negative thoughts can rapidly crowd our mind – if we allow them to. Next time this happens to you, create a mantra, something that you can repeat over and over, such as your goal statement: 'I will lose 9 kg (20 lb) in weight. I will lose 9 kg (20 lb) in weight.' By repeatedly saying a phrase like this, you are not giving negative thoughts a chance to creep in and alter your behaviour.

Negative thoughts in your head are best discarded before they corrode all the good work you have put in place when setting your goals. Overriding them with positive statements will help put you up there with successful dieters, who have taken a step change in their eating habits, lost weight – and kept it off.

AND I SAY TO MYSELF – WHAT A WONDERFUL WORLD

Equally, positive thoughts can play a big part in your thinking and behaviour. Repeating your positive mantra keeps it in the forefront of your consciousness and helps rid yourself of negativity. Well thought-out diets don't fail – dieters allow themselves to lapse; it is they who fail. Your success is perfectly controllable and is always in your hands.

NOW – PREPARE FOR SUCCESS

You have now set yourself up for success. By setting your goals using creative visualisation, your mind and body thinks that your objectives have already been achieved. You will start to act and talk differently, and more positively. Of course some readers may still think that this mind-over-matter stuff is complete nonsense – until they do it for themselves and discover that it really does work. Make this work for yourself and you will never look back; creative visualisation will become an everyday part of your continuing success.

The art of visualising your future success is arguably the single most powerful self-development tool that you can use when starting a diet or health plan.

CHAPTER 7

GETTING PREPARED
FOR THE DIET

Changing the way you eat and drink is rarely an easy or instant adjustment. You have to establish a new routine for yourself, a daily pattern that feels comfortable. Like following a recipe, it's best to read the ingredients and method (what you need to have and do) in advance. This way you can set your home up to help, not hinder you, and you can start getting into the right frame of mind.

MEASURE YOURSELF
AND SET YOUR GOALS

It's good to know where you are starting from so that you have a good record of your success. If you are setting a target weight for a specific date, like a wedding or holiday, expect to lose on average 0.5–1.0 kg (1–2 lb) a week.

When you weigh yourself it's best to do it at the same time of day and ideally naked, so there are no fluctuations caused by what you have been eating or the clothes you wear. First thing in the morning is good – often your lightest time of the day.

CALCULATE YOUR BMI
(BODY MASS INDEX)

BMI is a measure of whether you are a healthy weight for your height. It is a medical calculation that gives you an indication of your risk of disease (such as heart disease, diabetes and some cancers) due to your weight, while taking your height into consideration. As a general rule, a BMI of 18.5 to 24.9 means you are a healthy weight for your height. A BMI of 25 to 29.9 is 'overweight' and 30 plus is 'obese'.[1]

Knowing your BMI when you are overweight can help you appreciate how important it is to take action and also be a good motivator to lose weight. Alternatively, you may find that although you feel overweight and have gained weight over the years, you are still within the 'healthy weight' range. This is reassuring from a health perspective, but only you know your preferred weight within this zone; the weight that feels and looks best for your build.

You can calculate your BMI on the various sites on the internet, and also download iPhone apps to calculate and track your BMI over time (see page 266).

Calculation: Weight (kg) divided by Height (m) squared

To give you an idea of how BMI works out in practice – see opposite the average height for a man and a woman in the UK and the weight you have to be to fall into each band.

	Underweight	Healthy weight	Overweight	Obese
Woman 1.6 m (5 ft 3 in)	47 kg (7 st 6 lb) or less	48 kg (7 st 7 lb) to 63.5 kg (10 st 0 lb)	64 kg (10 st 1 lb) to 76.5 kg (12 st 1 lb)	77 kg (12 st 2 lb) or more
Man 1.75 m (5 ft 9 in)	56.5 kg (8 st 13 lb) or less	57 kg (9 st 0 lb) to 76 kg (12 st 0 lb)	76.5 kg (12 st 1 lb) to 91 kg (14 st 6 lb)	91.5 kg (14 st 7 lb) or more

WAIST TO HIP RATIO

If you are overweight, your health could be at greater risk, depending on where the extra body fat is stored. We store spare body fat under the skin, and also around the vital organs in our abdomen. It has been found that people with more fat around their abdomen (known as 'apple' shaped) are at more risk than 'pear' shaped people, who have more weight around their bottom and thighs.

The waist to hip ratio assesses the amount of fat deposited in your abdomen. The higher the ratio, the more fat is stored in your abdomen, and the more you are at risk from diseases linked to obesity, such as heart disease and diabetes.

HOW TO CALCULATE WAIST TO HIP RATIO

Using a metric tape measure:

1 measure your hips – at the widest point of your buttocks (cm);

2 measure your waist – at the narrowest point, usually just above your belly button (cm);

3 divide the waist number by the hip number.

A ratio of 1.0 or more in men or 0.85 or more in women indicates that you are an 'apple' shape carrying too much weight around your middle, and it's particularly important that you take action to lose weight. Try to get that ratio down below these figures.

KEEPING A FOOD DIARY

Before you start your diet it can help to keep a food diary, recording everything you eat and drink for at least three days. This gives you a good impression of where and when your weak spots are and will help you prepare strategies to avoid them. It's also nice to look back on your first food diary once you have lost some weight and notice how much your eating habits have changed since you started following the Mount Athos Diet.

RECORD YOUR PROGRESS

Make a good record of all your initial measurements and make this the beginning of a diary designed to track what you are doing and your progress while following the diet. While not wanting anyone to become obsessive about a diet, it can be really motivating to see your progress (or spur you into action if you have relaxed your approach).

Keep a weekly note of your weight (the same time and day each week), how much exercise you are doing, and notes on recipes that worked well for you. This will help you to see patterns and learn from your good and bad experiences. A greater understanding of your eating habits is the best way to ensure you tackle them and make a change, long term.

CLEAR THE HOUSE OF TEMPTATION

Before starting your diet it's a good idea to empty the house of less healthy food and drinks. Out of sight, out of mind really can help, so ditch or donate what you don't want to have around any more. If you know your weakness is late-night biscuit eating, just make sure there aren't any in your cupboards. You are less likely to make a special trip to the shops to stock up if you remember your original motivation in throwing them out in the first place.

If you have a house full of people to feed as well as yourself, try to gradually change the kitchen to become a healthy space for all the family. It's better for everyone to have less opportunity to snack on unhealthy foods and drinks, and you can always buy treats when you are out, rather than having them at home.

If you want to avoid cooking different meals on Fast Days, it's possible to share the same dishes with the rest of the family. To make them a bit more substantial for others who aren't trying to lose weight, and children, you can add some more of the starchy foods (like bread or pasta) as well as extra cheese, eggs or meat.

LEARN TO COOK AND EAT IN A BETTER, HEALTHIER WAY

To create tasty low-fat, no-meat meals for Fast Days, you will probably need to learn some new recipes and techniques in the kitchen. If you have never eaten as a vegetarian or vegan, it might take a little time to get used to not having meat, fish or chicken as the centrepiece of a meal. You can start trying out some of the recipes before you begin the diet properly (see pages 133–186) and have a look through Chapter 8 (pages 67–75) for more ideas on how to approach the diet.

STOCK UP ON THE FOODS YOU NEED TO SUCCEED

Read through the diet plan (see page 37) and work out what you need to buy. Think about the recipes that appeal to you for Fast Days and Moderation Days and get the ingredients you need (see Chapter 10 for more tips on a healthy store-cupboard). We have offered a range of recipes for Fast Days to give you the flexibility to create something very simple and quick when time is limited, as well as some more complex dishes with additional ingredients.

CHECK YOUR KITCHEN EQUIPMENT

The Mount Athos Diet is not an expensive diet to follow; in fact, it's more likely to save you money, but there a couple of pieces of kitchen equipment that are worth investing in if you don't have them already.

A good **medium-sized non-stick pan** with a well-fitting lid will help you prepare lots of dishes, including soups and stews with the minimum amount of fat needed. A good-quality non-stick frying pan is also useful for frying vegetables like onions, tomatoes and courgettes, as well as simple stir-fried veg, in almost no fat (see Chapter 9 for more tips on low-fat cooking).

The other invaluable piece of equipment is a **stick blender**. These simple hand-held blenders make it easy to produce great home-made soups (as well as smooth sauces, milkshakes and lots more). The basic ones are very reasonably priced.

Also, check the size of your crockery. If your dinner plates are really big, make sure you have a **smaller plate** to use on Fast Days, so you will be less likely to overdo it on your portion sizes.

PLANNING YOUR DIET PATTERN

You need to plan three Fast Days into your week. Monday, Wednesday and Friday is the easiest pattern and the one followed by the monks. The diet is flexible though, and you can pick the days that best suit your regular routine (although it's best if you can fast on intermittent days rather than three consecutive days). We have also found that the more regular your pattern of Fast Days, the easier it is to follow. Look through your calendar to see when celebrations or activities are planned, and make sure you work out when to Feast and when to Fast.

CHAPTER 8

TIPS FOR ACHIEVING SUCCESS ON THE DIET

DRINK PLENTY OF WATER

It's a good idea to be well hydrated when you are on a diet, eating less than usual. Get into the habit of drinking water regularly through the day so you don't mistake thirst for hunger. Some research suggests that drinking more water while you are dieting can help you lose more weight.[1] The scientific evidence for this is limited, but it's good to drink water regularly anyway, and it won't do you any harm. Two litres (3½ pints) a day is a good rule of thumb, although you will be drinking more in the summer months.

DIET DRINKS AREN'T THE ANSWER

If you are trying to lose weight, it goes without saying that you should stop drinking sweet fizzy drinks like colas, energy drinks and sports drinks. They are all loaded with sugar – just lots of calories with no nutritional benefit. So you may be thinking that you will swap them for the diet alternatives, rather than water, as they also contain no sugar. But if you want to lose weight and keep the weight off, it's better not to turn to drinks containing artificial sweeteners for two reasons. Firstly there's evidence that they may actually lead to eating more than you usually do, and secondly they do nothing to help you reduce your sweet tooth.

Diet drinks might seem to be a healthy alternative to the sugar-packed originals (there are a shocking 8 teaspoons of sugar in a 330 ml (11 fl oz) can of cola), but there are increasing concerns that when drunk regularly they may actually make you gain weight, and increase your risk of diseases like heart disease, stroke and diabetes. These risks seem to be similar in people who drink diet drinks as those drinking the regular ones.

This feels counter-intuitive, as the calorie and sugar content is much lower in diet drinks, but research from human and animal studies suggests that the artificial sweeteners in these drinks confuse the body's natural ability to manage calories based on tasting something sweet.

Artificial sweeteners are tricksters. First, they trick your taste buds into thinking that you are consuming sugar – that's why they taste sweet. Then, they fool and confuse your digestive and metabolic systems, and undermine the unconscious processes that help us regulate our weight and blood sugar. While in our conscious minds, artificial sweeteners can also create 'cognitive distortions', meaning we can fall into the trap of thinking a piece of cake is okay because we're having it with a diet drink. So, through both physiological and psychological effects, consuming artificial sweeteners can make you more likely to eat more than you would normally.[2]

Diet drinks are better than regular ones for your teeth, but in the long run they are not helping you to consume less sugar and curb your calorie intake. A sweet tooth is learnt and, therefore, can be changed. The less sweet things you eat and drink, the less you need to eat to create a sense of 'sweetness' (the same goes for salt). So it's better to get used to eating and drinking less sweet things, rather than looking for sweet alternatives. Water is more refreshing, it's not processed (so has a lower carbon footprint than a diet drink) ... and it's what a monk would drink.

SOUP FILLS YOU UP

Monks eat lots of soups and light stews on Fast Days, and it's a good idea for you, too. Studies have shown that soups can help you feel fuller for longer. It seems that it's more about the water being mixed with the food, than just having the extra water. One study measured how long people felt 'satiated' after eating a solid meal with a glass of water, compared with consuming the same amount of food and water as a soup. The group who had the soup didn't start to feel hungry again until a whole hour later than the other group.[3]

This means that soups are a good strategy for Fast Days when you are consuming fewer calories. It's worth making your own, though, to ensure they are low fat, packed with vegetables, and aren't loaded with salt (see the recipe section on pages 145–157 for lots of ideas).

BECOME AWARE OF 'ENERGY DENSITY'

Energy density is the amount of calories in a set weight of food. Fat and sugar in foods and drinks increase energy density, while more water, fruit and vegetables effectively dilute the energy density of a food or meal, making it lower. This is another way of thinking about the calorie content of foods.

The Mount Athos Diet is not about counting calories: it's about the food itself. It's helpful to be aware of the number of calories in unhealthy snacks, desserts and drinks as it can help motivate you to say 'no', and avoid them. Did you know that a slice of banoffee pie could contain up to 395 calories, a portion of chips up to 425 calories and a Mars Bar 260 calories? Understanding which foods are loaded with calories (and are energy dense) will help you save these treats for your Feast Days, and not let them jeopardise your Fast Day efforts.

When you are eating less food to lose weight, you want the food you eat to be nutrient dense, rather than energy dense, containing as many of the valuable nutrients that you need every day. Sweet, fatty foods contain a lot of 'empty calories' (calories without the nutrients), giving you another reason to do your best to avoid them. You will get the best nutrition from wholefoods and meals cooked from scratch at home using real ingredients.

Check the nutrition information on food packaging to find out how many calories are in a portion of any food you are tempted to eat. You might be surprised.

DON'T EAT LATE AT NIGHT

Our body is hardwired not to have food at night, but people now eat for more hours of the day and spend less hours 'fasting' at night. Historically, we used to only eat during the day over a 10–12 hour period, but now, with our social lives starting after sunset, it's gone up to a period of 16–18 hours a day.

Some research is beginning to show that it may not just be *what* you eat, but also *when* you eat that affects how easily you lose weight. Research into circadian rhythm (our 24-hour body clock) has established that the liver and stomach digest food and burn up fat more effectively during the day rather than at night, and, more and more, concerns about the effect our non-stop eating habits are having on our health are beginning to emerge, particularly in relation to obesity and diabetes.

On a practical level, when following a diet it makes sense to only eat during the day and avoid snacking into the night. Having your evening meal early will also help you to reduce early evening cravings. On a Fast Day you should be feeling a bit hungry when you go to bed – this is a good sign, so embrace it.

PORTION SIZES

Over recent years there has been a significant increase in the portion sizes available in fizzy drinks, snack foods, takeaways and restaurant meals. Combine this with the abundance of 'buy one, get one free' deals – often for sugary, fatty foods – and it is easy to overeat, without always noticing it. This super-sizing of our food has been recognised as a problem in our modern relationship with food, especially as we are much less active than we were just two generations ago. Most of us eat far more than we require for our energy needs when confronted by larger portions.

Here are ten tips for enjoying smaller portions:

1 use smaller plates;
2 only serve a volume of food that you could cup in both hands;
3 sit down to eat, turn off the television, shut that book and concentrate; distractions tempt us to eat mindlessly;

4 slow down and chew every mouthful. Savour and enjoy your food;

5 put your knife and fork down after each mouthful;

6 don't immediately go for that second helping. Wait for 10 minutes – do you still want it? It takes that time for your body to register 'fullness';

7 after serving, put any leftovers away from temptation;

8 drink water with your meal;

9 share restaurant dishes; one between two is often sufficient (and very cost-effective), or order a smaller portion (have a starter size for your main meal);

10 make a note of what you have eaten and write it down in a daily logbook.

BREAK THE SNACKING HABIT

Opportunities to eat are everywhere: the corner shop, the coffee shop, fast food joints, vending machines. If you have some money in your pocket you need never feel hungry. It's no surprise that the foods and drinks we consume between meals have become a significant part of the obesity problem across the West. They can add a serious load to calorie intake, usually with minimum nutritional value.

Most of us are lucky enough to have forgotten what being truly hungry feels like and instead we generally feel satisfied most of the time, eating as soon as any pang of hunger appears. If you are skinny or have an active job, then this might be fine, but for most people this is extra calories that you don't need. Monks, like most people one or two generations ago, rarely snack. They don't eat between meals, only at appointed meal times – and you should aim for this, too.

If you are a snacker then you will need to change your habits, both in terms of how often you reach for a snack and what you choose to nibble when you do. Know your weak moments and break the cycle. Think about when you are most likely to snack and what you could do to avoid it. Is it mid-morning at work, or on the way home? While you are cooking dinner, or watching television? Know yourself and work out your strategies, while at the same time try to start embracing hunger as a positive feeling.

Hunger can feel urgent between meals, but if you try to distract yourself with something else and keep busy, you will find that the feeling passes after about half an hour. Recognise the feeling and know that nothing bad will happen if you ignore it. Find something to do when you might normally give in to peckish moments. If you always have a biscuit with a cup of tea, try a different sort of drink for a while to see if that helps break the rut. If you really feel the need to eat something between meals, have a piece of fresh fruit, or a couple of small pieces of dried fruit (such as figs, dates, apricots, etc.), a few nuts or a plain cracker.

If you want to snack for emotional reasons – you are bored, fed up, stressed or frustrated – then try to distract yourself. If this happens to you a lot, it might be worth making a list of things that you can do when you reach for food but aren't really hungry. It could be calling a friend, doing a puzzle, looking at photos, ironing, putting on a good song. Think about what's best for you. Giving yourself half an hour can also work well in this case. If you find that you can't stop yourself, just get back on the wagon the next day, and be a bit stricter with yourself on the next Moderation Day.

REDUCE THE RISK OF TEMPTATION

Out of sight, out of mind … It's common sense that if you want to eat less of something, it's best not to have it around you, within easy access. At weak, bored, tired moments the temptation might just be too strong. You don't want to be faced with something you shouldn't eat every time you open your kitchen cupboard as that requires more willpower than should be necessary. So it's best not to buy unhealthy snacks and drinks. If you do need to have them in the house for others, then put them in a less obvious place where you won't regularly see them.

EXPAND YOUR RECIPE REPERTOIRE

Most people have a limited number of recipes they cook most often. It might not be the same meal on the same day of the week, every week, which used to be common, but it's likely that you have a certain number of recipes that you can cook effortlessly, without thinking. When you start a new way of eating as with the Mount Athos Diet, you will need to adopt a few extra recipes.

We suggest finding a range of Fast Day recipes that suit you, your tastes and your home situation and get used to cooking them. You may have to follow a recipe carefully a few times, but after a while it will become second nature and the effort needed will be minimal. Likewise, look at family favourites and see whether they can be adapted to suit the requirements of a Fast Day.

Soups or stews can be made in batches and frozen to heat up on Fast Days through the week. This will make it easier if you also have to cook different food for others in the family.

PLAN YOUR FAST DAYS

The Mount Athos Diet is flexible and you can work it around your regular pattern of life, as well as make occasional exceptions when special events occur. Aim to fast on intermittent days rather than three days in a row, for example, the monks at Mount Athos fast on Mondays, Wednesdays and Fridays. The beauty of the diet, however, is its flexibility to adapt to your lifestyle and allow for the unexpected things that can scupper the best-laid plans ...

Choose your Fast Days carefully, as it's easier to avoid snacking and temptation when you are busy. Distraction is a great help, so plan your Fast Days with this in mind. Work days might be best if you are at an office – busy with little opportunity to snack when the mood takes you.

CHAPTER 9

COOKING PRINCIPLES FOR THE DIET

To follow the Mount Athos Diet, you will probably need to adapt one or more of your cooking habits. As well as learning how to create more plant-based meals on Fast Days, you also need to cook with less fat. In this chapter we cover some key techniques to help you achieve this.

EXPLORE DIFFERENT CUISINES

The majority of recipes that we have included in this book are Mediterranean in style. But as many vegetarians know, when you are trying to eat less meat and fish, you need to look to a broad range of cuisines to build up your repertoire of delicious, as well as healthy, plant-based meals. Learn from the best cuisines that feature many vegetarian dishes, such as Indian, Far Eastern, Middle Eastern and South American, as well as the Mediterranean.

Vegetarian dishes in these regions have usually developed for reasons of religious vegetarianism or poverty. Meat and fish are expensive, so peasant food is often vegetarian, with maybe a small amount of meat added. As well as using the recipes in this book, search your cookbooks or the internet for vegetarian and vegan recipes. You will find that many of them can be adapted to use minimal oil for Fast Day meals, and you will also find that they give you ideas for flavour combinations you may not have tried before.

COOKING WITH MINIMAL FAT

Some cooking methods naturally require no additional oil or fat, such as poaching, steaming, grilling or using a tagine. For dishes that begin with a dash of oil in a pan, there are a couple of different ways to overcome this or to reduce the quantity of oil required. A non-stick pan can be used to 'dry-fry' onions or similar; if food begins to catch on the base of the pan, a small amount of water can help to keep things moving.

Another option is to use an oil spray. These are available to buy ready-made, or you could make your own using a clean spray bottle filled with five parts oil to one part water. Just a spray or two on the base of the pan before use will be enough. Similarly, you could try using a pastry brush to brush a thin layer of oil on the base of the pan before placing on the heat. Cooking over a low heat with the lid on will preserve any water that would be lost, and effectively helps to 'steam-fry' the vegetables in the pan.

Soups and stews can often be adapted to cook ingredients in the cooking liquid from the start, without frying any of the ingredients beforehand. Many curries begin life this way, such as the Lentil Dal on page 170.

HERBS AND SPICES

When cooking with minimal oil and minimal salt, especially on Fast Days, you need to add flavour from elsewhere. Herbs and spices bring life to recipes that can otherwise be quite dull, so try recipes from different cuisines to help you explore many different flavour combinations.

Fresh herbs, particularly, are an easy way to make a significant difference to a meal, so get used to using them and be quite generous with the amounts you add. Fresh herbs can be quite expensive to buy, so it's worth growing some on the windowsill, patio or in the garden. Mint, thyme, sage, oregano, rosemary, basil and chives are all very easy to grow. Coriander and parsley are worth buying in pots from the supermarket, as you can snip off the amount you need as you go.

ADDING DRESSINGS

Dressings are one of the hardest condiments to get right when dieting. A classic French dressing uses two parts oil to one part vinegar, and it's difficult to find a good substitute when working with this ratio. Shop-bought low-cal dressings are full of sugar or sweeteners, so it's always best to make your own. On Fast Days, the best thing to use is the simplest: a good squeeze of fresh lemon or lime juice, or a splash of balsamic vinegar (a white balsamic won't colour the salad).

On Moderation Days, make use of one of Greece's best-known exports: Greek yogurt. As well as the many health benefits of good, natural yogurt, it's a versatile food that can be easily adapted to create a multitude of sauces including dressings. For example, blend 250 g (9 oz) of Greek yogurt with a couple of roasted peppers for a tasty salad topping. This type of sauce can be used in many recipes that specify a swirl of cream.

USING SLOW COOKERS

Slow cookers are a good way to keep in the flavour and texture of meat or fish, which makes them perfect for warming stews. Slow cookers are also particularly convenient for those who work outside the home. A small amount of preparation in the morning and you could come home to a delicious meal ready and waiting for you in the evening.

Liquid levels can be tricky to get right when using a slow cooker, as vegetables tend to lose a lot of their liquid while cooking, so when converting from traditional recipes to slow cooker equivalents you will need to reduce the amount of liquid required. If in doubt, use a recipe designed specifically for this way of cooking.

EATING SOUP

As mentioned in Chapter 8, soup is a dieter's best friend. Filling, versatile and delicious, there is no end to the combination of flavours achievable with a home-made soup. If you'd like to have a go at making up your own recipe, these tips may help you succeed.

- The cornerstone of many of the soups we enjoy in the West is the sautéed onion, cooked (until soft but not brown) in oil or fat. Classic French or Italian recipes often combine onions with finely chopped celery, carrot and garlic, and sometimes parsley, which is then cooked slowly. This forms a base that is rich and flavoursome. Adapt soup recipes to include the minimum of fat using the tips above.

- Other ingredients are then added, such as the types of vegetables that take a while to cook, but which add bulk and texture.
- Stock is a flavoured liquid, beginning life as water cooked with other ingredients to create a rich and tasty broth. Stock is added to the soup ingredients to add further flavour, layering up the dimensions of your dish. If time is tight a quality stock cube or bouillon powder is a good basis for the stock in a soup.
- Once the stock has been added, the soup then undergoes its main cooking period. The core vegetables should be simmered until just tender, at which point the soup can be blended if desired, or left as is (with distinct ingredients and more translucent broth).
- Either way, this is the point to add quick-cooking vegetables, tiny soup pasta shapes, cheese or cooked meat or fish, just to quickly cook them (vegetables or pasta) or bring them up to temperature.
- Some soups benefit from a topping: crunchy seeds, a swirl of silky yogurt, croûtons, chunks of cheese or fresh herbs. This is a good time to experiment: a soup topping can elevate this simple dish to something special.
- Other cuisines approach soup-making differently, with many of the Far Eastern recipes bypassing the onion-softening stage, instead combining base ingredients with the stock and cooking without fat. This is a useful tip as it means Fast Day soups can be even lighter (for example, the Japanese Noodle Soup, page 149). You can also try other kinds of soups without the frying stage, such as the Mount Athos Bean and Lentil Soups (pages 155 and 154).

TAGINE COOKING

Tagines are used throughout Morocco to cook quick and very flavourful food. The cooking pot – the tagine – consists of a circular dish with a groove around its top on which sits a separate, close-fitting conical lid. The food cooked in it is also known as a tagine.

Tagine pots come in many sizes, serving anything from two to eight people. They are usually made from either terracotta, glazed or unglazed, or with a cast-iron base. The terracotta tagine goes in the oven while the cast-iron version cooks on the hob.

This one-pot cooking system could not be simpler. As the food starts to cook steam rises within the conical lid and condenses, dripping down the interior into the shallow groove in which it sits. This puddles and forms a seal, so the food not only cooks from the base of the pot – it steams. And it is the steam that cooks the food so rapidly; a chicken tagine will be ready in 20 minutes.

We find cooking in a cast-iron based tagine more flexible as they can be used in the oven or on the hob. If you don't possess a tagine, substitute an ordinary wide-based, lidded saucepan; close the lid tightly when cooking by placing a sheet of foil over the pan before putting the lid on. This will ensure that most of the steam given off stays in the pan.

Assembling a tagine meal is very easy. Ingredients only need to be cut appropriately – tougher meats cut smaller, vegetables and fish larger.

Moroccan food is highly spiced. Typical spices which feature a lot in Moroccan and Tunisian cuisine include cinnamon, cardamom seeds, cumin, turmeric, star anise, ginger, caraway, cayenne pepper, paprika (plain or smoked), coriander and saffron. An alternative to sourcing several different spices is to use Ras el hanout – a classic blend of North African spices.

The heat in tagines is usually supplied by the ubiquitous multi-spice paste – harissa. Raisins, dates or figs are also regularly added to savoury meat dishes. (See pages 165, 200 and 202 for some delicious vegetable, fish and chicken tagine recipes.)

CHAPTER 10

FOODS TO ENJOY ON THE MOUNT ATHOS DIET

The Mount Athos Diet includes a broad range of plant-based foods for you to enjoy. The lack of animal protein might seem like the biggest challenge to overcome; it is far from being the norm in terms of the way we eat in the Western world, but don't be discouraged; it's actually a very healthy way to eat, as many other parts of the world agree. Vegan, vegetarian or carnivore, finding plenty of plant proteins is easier than you think.

As some of these foods may be new to you, what follows is a run-down of some of the tastiest beans, pulses, grains, nuts and seeds, and other 'superfoods', and how to use them in your cooking. Once you have cooked with them a few times, you will have the confidence to be a bit more adventurous and begin experimenting with your own combinations.

BEANS AND PULSES

Pulses are underused in the UK. Although the nation loves baked beans, we are less enthusiastic about those other beans and pulses used daily in other cultures. Cheap to buy, this food group is a great way to feel fuller for longer, and they have the added benefit of absorbing flavour really well. It's no surprise that many curries feature beans and pulses, as they lend themselves as a vehicle for holding huge depth of flavour.

Though cheaper to soak and cook from scratch, this isn't always practical and so we suggest canned alternatives in the Mount Athos Diet recipes. If you do wish to soak and cook your own beans, please make sure you follow the instructions on the packet carefully so you do not become unwell.

Red split lentils – good for soups, dals and making into a smooth paste for dips or to add bulk to tomato sauces for pasta. On their own, red split lentils don't have a huge amount of flavour, but where they excel is in building texture as they break down when cooked. Plus, they carry flavours of herbs and spices well. Try the Lentil Dal on page 170.

Puy lentils – where red split lentils can be cooked down to a thick paste, Puy lentils are quite different. With an almost meaty flavour, these little blue/green lentils hold their shape very well. They are ideal for chunkier stews, as a tasty addition to salads, or in combination with fresh herbs, particularly thyme or bay leaves, as in the Braised Puy Lentils with Bay Leaves on page 172.

Green lentils – these are larger than red split lentils and Puy lentils, with a flavour and texture falling somewhere between the two. They are great for use in curries or soups, such as the Mount Athos Lentil Soup on page 154.

Chickpeas – the basis of hummus, these larger pulses have a great texture and flavour. Versatile and cheap, chickpeas can be found in many different types of food, from Italian pasta dishes to Indian curries. Chickpeas go particularly well with spinach, as well as tomatoes. Try the Moroccan Carrot and Chickpea Soup on page 145, the Hearty Harissa Salad on page 140, the Turkish Spiced Chickpea Soup on page 151 or the Moroccan Chickpea and Squash Stew on page 161.

Butter beans – large white beans with a nice soft texture, butter beans also hold their shape well. They are good for stews, salads and in pasta dishes, and their trademark dish is the Greek Baked Butter Beans (see page 167). Mashed, butter beans take on a texture close to mashed potato, as in the White Bean Mash on page 180.

Red kidney beans – the classic firm, red bean that takes centre-stage in the classic chilli con carne. Red kidney beans work well in stews, and can also be mashed to make the beginnings of a bean burger. Try the Mount Athos Bean Soup on page 155.

White beans – there are a number of different white beans available, including haricot (the classic baked bean) and cannellini, which are both good in salads, soups and casseroles. The Simple Bulgur Wheat Supper (page 179), White Bean Mash (page 180), Mackerel Salad (page 195) and the Thai-style Bean Patties (page 206) all contain haricot or cannellini beans.

Black beans – living up to their name, these are small dark beans and are packed with flavour. Not to be mistaken for black-eyed beans, black beans are a staple in Latin American and Mexican cuisine, forming the basis of refried beans and many a chilli recipe, such as the Black Bean Chilli on page 163.

Tofu

Tofu, also known as bean curd, is made from soya beans and originates from the Far East. It's a high quality protein alternative to meat, and though it is a rather bland ingredient, it can be transformed into a flavour-packed food with the addition of plenty of spices. Tofu will soak up a marinade or you can buy ready-flavoured versions, which come smoked or spiced (and some of these are even good enough to eat raw, and can be added to salads).

Plain tofu is available in several different textures: firm, soft or 'silken', and is usually sold packed in water. Drain and press between layers of kitchen paper before using, particularly if you want to fry it. Silken tofu can be made into sweet dishes, such as a vegan cheesecake, or blended to make vegan dips or pâtés. Freeze and defrost firm tofu before using, for a more chewy texture.

NUTS AND SEEDS

Nuts and seeds are a great way to add flavour and crunch to a dish, and they are nutrient packed. They are also a great source of protein, but be aware that they are also high in fat, although the fats they contain are generally the healthier unsaturated ones, but it's best not to go overboard. They make a good alternative to meat in meals on Fast Days, but if you snack on nuts, keep quantities small – no more than a small handful.

Scattered over a salad or ground and stirred into a sauce, the flavour and texture of nuts and seeds means a little goes a long way. Try making your own muesli, combining a few different types of nuts and seeds within it. And when cooking try lightly toasting nuts and seeds in a dry pan or in the oven to intensify their flavour even further.

Cashews – little 'c'-shaped nuts, cashews go well in stir-fries and Asian dishes instead of meat. Add them early on in the cooking so they soften nicely.

Walnuts – used frequently in French dishes, walnuts go well with blue cheese and pears. They add crunch and flavour when chopped and sprinkled over salads.

Almonds – ground or whole, almonds are a great way to add texture to a dish. Ground almonds can also be used in baking as a replacement or enriching ingredient to wheat flour, and a handful of toasted, flaked almonds adds another dimension to Middle Eastern stews.

Brazil nuts – with their mild, rich flavour, Brazil nuts are often used in baking. They also work well in a nut burger or a nut loaf roughly chopped.

Hazelnuts – while the classic pairing is with chocolate, hazelnuts also work well with chicken, white fish and avocado, and they make a great topping for salads.

Pistachios – little green nuts, pistachios are famous for the colour they give pistachio ice cream. They add flavour and texture to many Middle Eastern dishes, added both during and after cooking.

Peanuts – the most popular nuts in the UK that aren't officially nuts at all. Botanically they are beans, but because of their high fat content they tend to be thought of as nuts. Peanuts feature in lots of cuisines around the world. When ground down to a paste they are used in sauces (such as satay) and stews and relishes, and when finely chopped added as a topping to a dish. Peanut butter is a useful sandwich filler on Fast Days, but spread it thinly.

Sesame seeds – high in calcium, sesame seeds are tiny but packed with goodness and flavour. Ground, they form the basis for tahini, the sesame seed paste used as an ingredient in hummus. Sesame oil is a staple ingredient in Far Eastern cooking, but used for flavour rather than as an oil, so add sparingly. Sesame seeds are worth toasting before you add them to salads for a richer flavour.

Pumpkin seeds – these green seeds are a versatile ingredient, and are used in both savoury and sweet dishes, raw and cooked. They work well in a salad, but also as a natural accompaniment to pumpkin dishes – as a topping for pumpkin soup or to add crunch to a pumpkin curry or stew.

Sunflower seeds – one of the most commonly available seeds, sunflower seeds are a mainstay of muesli, cereal bars and other health food shop staples. Add them to a home-made stuffing mix for Mediterranean vegetables such as peppers, courgettes and tomatoes to add texture and flavour.

Pine nuts – a key ingredient in pesto, pine nuts are a Mediterranean and Middle Eastern cookery essential. Not technically a nut, pine nuts work well in pasta dishes and salads, such as the Roast Peppers, Spinach and Orange Salad on page 142.

GRAINS

Pearl barley – this makes a delicious soft and chewy addition to soups and stews. It's also suitable to use as an alternative to rice in risotto dishes.

Couscous – this is not actually a grain but is, in fact, tiny pieces of dried pasta made from wheat. It originates from North Africa and is traditionally served hot with stews and tagines, but is also delicious cold in salads.

Bulgur wheat – a great alternative to couscous, bulgur wheat has a firmer, slightly chewier texture and a mildly nutty flavour. It comes in various grades from fine to coarse, and forms the basis of the Middle Eastern salad dish, taboulleh. Try the Spicy Bulgur Wheat and Pea Pilaf (page 178) or the Simple Bulgur Wheat Supper on page 179.

Oats – one of the oldest and most used cereals, oats are packed with healthy, slow-release energy, making porridge a great breakfast option. Try the Bircher Muesli Breakfast Pot on page 187 or Stewed Apple with Oats (see page 133).

Quinoa – pronounced 'keen-wah', quinoa is the most protein-heavy plant on the planet. A versatile food, it's often cooked as a grain and served as an accompaniment, although you can also find it flaked or popped in breakfast cereals or protein bars. The Quick Quinoa Pilaf on page 174 is a good introduction to this nutritious grain.

Rice – brown, basmati, or wild, rice is a staple food, with much of the world eating rice dishes daily. White rice has had its outer coating removed, making it more processed and less nutritious than brown or wild rice. Brown rice is less processed and takes a little longer to cook, but has a nice firm texture and adds a nuttier flavour to a meal. Wild rice is actually a different variety of plant to Asian rices and is a particularly high-protein grain.

DAIRY, FISH AND MEAT

When you do eat dairy, fish or white meat on Moderation Days, and if you have meat on Feast Days your portions should be modest, and are likely to be smaller than what you ate before the diet. We urge you to choose carefully and think about quality over quantity. Rather than eat a big serving of animal protein from a questionable source, the Mount Athos Diet advocates small portions of better quality produce.

As well as supporting good practice in the food industry, the culinary and psychological implications of buying well but eating less can't be ignored. A small, organically farmed chicken bought from a local supplier will have more flavour than its battery-farmed equivalent, and its provenance will encourage you to cook it well and savour every mouthful.

VEGETABLES

Aim to eat a variety of different types of vegetables, of different colours: that way you will be getting a wide range of all the beneficial phytochemicals that are so good for you, in addition to all the vitamins and minerals. Always look for ways to get more veggies into your meals, so whip up a side salad to have with a soup, or throw whatever bits and bobs you can find in the refrigerator into the wok for a nifty stir-fry. The more vegetables the better; it goes back to the energy and nutrient-dense foods we discussed in Chapter 8 – basically, it's better to fill up on the foods that contain less calories that are also packed with nutrients.

Vegetable box delivery schemes are a great way to ensure regular supplies of well produced, reasonably priced, seasonal produce, and can help you to become more adventurous in your cooking.

Potatoes – jacket potatoes are a dieter's friend when served in moderate-sized portions and without butter or oil. Wash, thread on to a metal skewer, and bake for an hour in an oven preheated to 180°C/350°F/Gas mark 4. Peeled and chopped, potatoes can be added to many dishes that allow for a cooking time of around 30 minutes, and floury potatoes act as a natural thickener in soups or stews.

Carrots – a versatile root vegetable, they can often improve a dish's depth. Experiment with different ways of preparing carrots: grate raw into a salad or add grated carrot to a stew halfway through cooking; or roast with other veg.

Green, leafy veg – spinach, kale and cabbage are often best eaten lightly cooked, and in some cases raw. Highly nutritious, not only are these vegetables tastier when lightly cooked, but this way they also have a higher vitamin count. Frozen leaf spinach is a decent frozen vegetable that's handy to have in reserve, and can be added to pasta dishes, curries and sauces.

Courgettes – easy to grow and simple to cook, courgettes are a great Mediterranean vegetable to make the most of during the summer months. Sliced, they work well in stir-fries, with pasta, or fried with a little oil and garlic. Larger courgettes can be stuffed with a tasty nut- or seed-based stuffing.

Aubergines – best cooked slowly with tomatoes, aubergines also work well as part of a vegetable bake. Charred under the grill, peeled and blended with yogurt, aubergines can also form a delicious sauce for a curry, or mashed with lemon juice and spices taste good as a dip. Diced aubergine can soak up a lot of oil during cooking, but you can avoid this if you cook them slowly in a non-stick pan over a low heat with the lid on – the steam cooks the aubergine with only the minimum of fat needed.

Broccoli – a highly nutritious vegetable, broccoli can be used in more adventurous ways than we usually attempt. Great with chilli and garlic, broccoli is a mainstay in Italian vegetable dishes, and works very well with pasta alongside olives or lemon.

Peas – a vegetable that is almost as good from frozen as it is fresh, peas are a super-quick and easy vegetable to cook. Surprisingly good with cheese, they feature in curries, salads and other dishes, often paired with herbs, such as mint, or with lemon.

Leeks – this mild-flavoured member of the onion family can be added to almost any dish that requires onions, and are a perfect addition to soups and stews. They are also delicious served as a side, when 'steam-fried' with a little garlic and fresh herbs.

FRUIT

Following government advice as well as the example of the monks of Mount Athos, it's good to eat lots of fruit and vegetables every day – at least five portions. Don't turn to juice as an easy way to achieve this. Fruit juice has been refined and processed, so it's better to have the whole fruit. We recommend just one small glass of juice a day if you want to drink it.

Don't limit the amount of fresh fruit you eat. If you find that sometimes you need to eat something between meals, choose fruit. It's hard to eat too much of it, so it is usually self-regulating in amount. As with vegetables, it's better to eat a range of different types of fruits, than lots of one type. Be more careful with dried fruit, limiting yourself to just a small handful a day.

CHAPTER 11

WHAT TO DRINK ON THE MOUNT ATHOS DIET

It's good to keep yourself well hydrated when following any diet: that way you won't mistake thirst for hunger.

DRINKS FOR FAST DAYS AND MODERATION DAYS

Water – you can't beat a glass of ice-cold water on a hot summer's day, and you need to train your taste buds to think like this all the time. If you don't already drink water regularly every day, then this is a good habit to get into. Tap, mineral or spring water are all good choices, so choose whatever you prefer.

- Keep a bottle of water in the fridge all the time, so it's always cold.
- At work, keep a bottle of water near you to remind you to drink.
- If you like fizzy drinks, try fizzy water. You can have it neat, with a dash of lemon or lime juice in it, or you can use it to make a longer drink from a small glass of

juice – this works well with orange juice, apple juice and grape juice.

Herbal and fruit teas – these make a good low-caffeine alternative to standard tea and coffee. Drink them straight with no sugar or milk to make them a perfect alternative to tea and coffee on Fast Days. You might find it easier to have a completely different drink instead of cutting the milk and sugar out of your standard tea and coffee.

Coffee/tea – you can drink tea and coffee in moderation, but limit yourself to only a few cups a day, so you don't overload on caffeine. Drink your tea and coffee without milk and sugar, and definitely avoid the large and indulgent drinks in coffee shops – extra syrup, cream or toppings will obviously push up the amount of calories significantly.

Don't turn diet drinks into a habit – you shouldn't drink sweet fizzy drinks on Fast or Moderation Days. It's also not a good idea to regularly swap them for diet, sugar-free versions. The odd one isn't a problem if you want to avoid a full-sugar drink, but see page 67 for reasons why it's not good to build artificial sweeteners into your routine.

Fruit juices and smoothies – it's fine to have small amounts of these drinks on Fast and Moderation Days, but avoid the ones with added sugar, and don't have too much of them. These juices are refined, so limit yourself to one small glass a day.

Alcohol – remember that like sugar, alcohol is empty calories – i.e. calories with no nutritional benefit. Avoid excess alcohol and drink only within the limits of the diet. If you drink regularly, it will make a big difference to your calorie intake when you cut down to this level. Following the intermittent fasting pattern of the Mount Athos Diet will mean that you can't drink alcohol for three days of the week. And on the three Moderation Days you should only be having two units of alcohol, preferably red wine. On the Feast Day you can have more if you want to.

The monks drink their home-made red wine with meals when they are not fasting. Research has suggested that small, regular amounts of red wine like this can reduce your risk of heart disease, so we recommend red wine on Moderation Days, and choose lower alcohol contents where you can.

Feast Days only – avoid these the rest of the week
- Sweet fizzy drinks, such as colas, orange drinks, lemonade, etc., as well as energy drinks and sports drinks.
- Cordials – such as orange squash, elderflower cordial.
- Calorie-packed coffees from coffee shops.
- Sweetened milkshakes.

CHAPTER 12

ALCOHOL AND THE DIET

Drinks range in alcohol content widely – in the broadest sense from spirits to beers for example. But then also within each category the number of units per drink can vary, and the size of your glass will also affect the number of units you consume in each drink. For this reason recommendations about alcohol and health are usually expressed in 'units'.

It's recommended that you shouldn't regularly exceed **2–3 units per day if you are a woman**, and **3–4 units per day if you are a man**. And after a heavy drinking session, you should avoid alcohol for 48 hours afterwards.

WHAT IS A UNIT?

A unit is 10 ml of pure alcohol. Alcoholic drinks are labelled with the percentage of pure alcohol in them. This might be expressed as for example 13%, or in many cases as 13 ABV (alcohol by volume). You can use this figure to compare the strength of different drinks, but it doesn't actually help you work out how many units you are drinking.

The alcohol content of many drinks has crept up slowly over the years, as have the sizes of the wine glasses. When the 'unit' concept was introduced, it was roughly equivalent to a half pint of weak beer, a small old-fashioned balloon-style glass of wine or one shot of spirit. Now with stronger beers, ciders, wines and numerous other 'alcopop' drinks available, together with a variety of glass sizes to choose from, it's not as easy to keep track of your units.

Fortunately, following pressure from the government, drinks companies are increasingly labelling the number of units per drink on bottles, making it easier to check how much you are drinking. Below are some examples of the number of units in different drinks. The Mount Athos Diet includes 2 units of alcohol, preferably red wine on Moderation Days. As you can see here, that is equivalent to one standard 175 ml (6 fl oz) glass of 12% wine. Like the monks, drink weaker varieties rather than the stronger (often New World) wines, and have your wine with a meal.

Wine:

1 small glass (125 ml/4 fl oz) 12% wine = 1.5 units
1 standard glass (175 ml/4 fl oz) 12% wine = 2.1 units
1 large glass (250 ml/9 fl oz) 12% wine = 3.0 units

A standard 750 ml bottle of 13.5% wine contains 10 units.

Beer:

1 pint (600 ml) 3.6% beer, lager or cider = 2 units
1 pint (600 ml) 5.2% beer, lager or cider = 3 units

Spirits:

1 single, small 25 ml (1 fl oz) shot 40% spirits = 1 unit

THE DANGERS OF DRINKING TOO MUCH

Although the monks' moderate way of life results in a low intake of wine, the Western world sees alcohol as a major concern, affecting our health, our weight and our wallets. This is especially true of Britain, one of the fattest nations in Europe and home to some of the biggest drinkers, too. Based on 2012 figures released by the UK's Office of National Statistics, medical experts forecast that 210,000 people will die from alcohol abuse in the next 20 years.

In addition to long-term effects, obesity and alcohol health problems go hand in hand. The average wine drinker consumes 2,000 extra calories a month, putting on a half a stone (3 kg/7 lb) of fat a year.

One glass of wine has a similar number of calories as a slice of cake. The calorie content of a full glass of beer is similar to a glass of single cream. You will need to run 15–20 minutes to burn them off. Cut down on alcohol and you will cut down on all those 'empty' calories too.

UNDERSTAND YOUR DRINKING AND MAKE CHANGES

Are you concerned about your relationship with alcohol and worried that you may be drinking too much? Take the drinking self-assessment and find out how many units you are drinking by visiting www.drinkaware.co.uk.

THE MERITS OF DRINKING RED WINE IN MODERATION

The monks drink red wine in moderation on four days of the week – a total of around 12 units maximum each per week and they only drink it with food. If you do drink, it's good to follow their example. Their limited intake of alcohol is regarded as one of several contributors to their longevity.

There is general agreement among scientists that there is something in red wine that, when drunk in moderation, can help to prevent blood clots, protect the heart and reduce 'bad' cholesterol. Lots of research is underway exploring what it is about red wine that is beneficial, and early contenders include tannins, some types of flavonols, and resveratrol, which is found in the skin of red grapes.

Several monasteries on Mount Athos have vineyards and produce their own wine. Three well-known Greek wines originate from Athos: Tsantali, Milopotamos and Monoxilitis.

CHAPTER 13

EATING OUT ON THE DIET

Eating out, whether in a restaurant or at a friend's house, can prove hazardous to the committed Mount Athos dieter. This is particularly true if you eat out several days in a week. The forced overindulgence can quickly threaten to derail your good intentions and earlier success.

When you eat out you are not in control of what goes into each dish. Unlike in someone's home, restaurants offer you choice, but they tend to use a lot of fat and it may not always be clear from the menu which dish is healthiest from the description.

When eating in a restaurant, scan the menu and notice which dishes follow the Mount Athos Diet principles. If there are none but some which come close, ask the waiter to delete certain elements and perhaps add more of others. Do your best to stick to the principles. It's hardest on Fast Days, but it's not the end of the word if you occasionally find yourself having to eat something that you weren't planning to. Just be stricter with yourself on the following Moderation Day.

WHEN EATING OUT IN A RESTAURANT

Restaurant portion sizes are often large so consider requesting a half portion (or starter-sized portion), or suggest sharing one plate with a fellow diner. On a Fast Day don't have a starter, just go straight to the main. As far as desserts go – fresh fruit is the only option, and in some restaurants this will be delicious – a bowl of strawberries or a fresh mango don't need anything else with them.

Here are some suggestions for when you eat out in different types of restaurants:

Pizza And Pasta Restaurants

A normal pizza – without cheese in the crust and such like – is a pretty healthy dish. Order carefully in these restaurants and you can easily stick to the Fast Day rules.

For example, you can choose:

- a vegetable-topped pizza and ask for no cheese on top;
- a simple tomato sauce with pasta – choose a small portion;
- a simple salad without an oily or creamy dressing. Dress your salad with vinegar only;
- or an Italian bean and vegetable soup as a main course.

Asian Restaurants

Noodle bars, Japanese, Chinese and Thai restaurants usually have light vegan dishes on the menu if you look carefully. There are rarely any dairy products in these cuisines, so you just need to look for vegetarian dishes, and choose a soup or a dish that isn't fried or in a rich sauce. If you are having rice with your meal, always order plain white rice.

Don't be tempted by fried starters, or foods in batter, whatever healthy-sounding ingredients may be in them. Try edamame beans if they are on the menu; they are a great healthy starter.

Some examples of what to choose:

- vegetarian sushi – filled with cucumber, tofu or avocado for example. Accompany with a seaweed salad;
- steamed vegetable dumplings;
- a vegetarian noodle soup, ideally with lots of vegetables in it;
- a mixed vegetable dish, with tofu or cashew nuts added.

Indian Restaurants

It's easy to find vegan dishes in Indian restaurants; the main issue is the amount of oil used in cooking. Avoid creamy curries like korma and pasanda, as well as fried starters such as bhajis or samosas. Stick to a simple combination of plain rice or chapatti with a dal or bean-based dish (ask the waiter which is lowest in fat), plus a vegetable dish or simple salad. Tandoori and madras curries tend to be lower in fat.

Kebab And Chip Shops

In lots of these takeaways it's hard to find anything suitable. Survey the menu as best you can. If you have to stray from the diet rules, eat the smallest portion. Fish and chip shops often serve rolls, a better choice than chips. And if you have a portion of fish – eat the fish but not the batter.

Kebab takeaways usually offer a greater range than chip shops, and on a Fast Day you can try hummus and salad in pitta bread – delicious and healthy. Falafels are made from chickpeas, but are deep-fried, so they are not a perfect choice, but are better than most of the other options on offer.

EATING SANDWICHES
WHEN OUT AND ABOUT

Ideally make your own sandwiches if you are not going to be home for lunch on a Fast Day, but if you do need to buy something out, it can be a challenge. You can sometimes find hummus sandwiches, and in an outlet where they make sandwiches fresh, a peanut butter sandwich might be possible. Alternatively, lots of the sandwich bars offer soups so choose a vegetarian one for a filling midday meal, or you may be able to find a bean- or grain-based salad.

OTHER OPTIONS WHEN EATING OUT

A jacket potato with baked beans (no butter or cheese) and a side salad is a great choice for a Fast Day. A selection of side dishes could be a delicious, vegetable-based option when there isn't much else on the menu.

GET THE NUTRITION INFORMATION

Several restaurant, fast food and coffee shop chains now supply the fat and calorie content of all the meals and drinks they sell. It may not always be easy to find it in the place itself, but many supply the information online if you want to check the best options before you go.

EATING WITH FRIENDS

Eating at a friend's house can present more hurdles, but you have the chance to contact them in advance to give them an idea of what you would like to eat. This is not always appropriate or possible, and you might not want to make a fuss in relation to your diet, so you may just have to think 'damage limitation' when you get there.

Most importantly, limit your portion sizes. Easy to do if you are serving yourself, though often you will have no choice and your meal will be plated up in the kitchen and brought directly to the table. If you are the first to be served and you feel that there is too much food on the plate, simply ask for less and say that you are following a very effective diet. Above all, do not be afraid of leaving food on your plate when you have finished your meal. You don't have to finish it. And no matter how tempting, don't go for seconds.

Desserts present more of an issue, as does drinking. Your host will want to treat you and most dinner parties are indulgent affairs. However, if you can be the designated driver you have a great excuse to abstain, and if you have been able to explain to your host about your diet then they should understand why you pass up the offer of dessert.

If all else fails, you may just need to pick up where you left off the next day, and incorporate an extra Fast Day into your week.

CHAPTER 14

EXERCISE, HEALTH AND THE MOUNT ATHOS DIET

Exercise alone will not make you slim, but it will help you stay slim as well as keeping you healthy; fitness and fundamental changes in your diet over the long term equal well-being.

Exercise is all about enhancing the ways our bodies work, but it's more than that. Although it's not possible to exercise your way to mental brilliance it is perfectly possible to exercise to happiness. Regular exercise brings with it many psychological benefits. Exercise releases chemicals called endorphins, which can trigger a positive lift in mood, boost self-esteem, ward off anxiety, reduce stress and improve sleep.

However, the expression 'There's no gain without pain' brings with it some truth. When we first start an exercise regime there can be a certain amount of pain (usually the first 30 minutes) to be endured before the euphoria kicks in. We are forcing our body to wake up from its slumber and initially this can prove an effort. But stick with it and your endorphins soon adopt their secondary role – that of blocking pain. Suddenly, this exercise thing seems to be getting a whole lot easier. Then, remarkably, you start to look forward to it.

Regular exercise and sensible eating combined help to ensure a healthy lifestyle. Failing to exercise places too much reliance on diet alone to achieve and maintain weight loss, especially as we get older when we tend to gain fat and lose muscle. Aerobic activity makes your body use more energy and by using more calories than you consume, you automatically aid weight loss. The key to enjoying the benefits of regular aerobic exercise and to sustaining behaviour change is to keep your exercise of choice simple, realistic and convenient. Choose an exercise regime that fits in with your life – what you can afford, where you live, and what free time you have.

Set yourself some realistic, measurable targets which you can enjoy achieving. Weekly goals are better than daily goals: they offer more flexibility and avoid feelings of guilt when for one reason or another it becomes difficult or impossible for you to exercise.

Write down your achievements; you will be surprised at how much they mount up. One of the authors logged their regular walks and clocked up an amazing time.

EXERCISE AND WEIGHT-LOSS MAINTENANCE

Exercise is of paramount importance in maintaining weight loss and ideally should be part of your daily/weekly regime. Research has shown that the only way to maintain weight loss is to be engaged in regular physical exercise.

The exact amount of exercise needed to maintain weight loss varies from person to person. Exercise alone will not help you maintain your weight loss – you must also maintain the Mount Athos Diet healthy eating plan.

HOW MUCH EXERCISE DO I NEED?

There is a lot of ill-informed advice and misinformation concerning exercise and weight loss. Here are the facts: a minimum average of 20–30 minutes' exercise a day will suffice. Both the UK's NHS (National Health Service) and the US Department of Health and Human Services recommend a minimum of 150 minutes' moderate aerobic exercise a week, or 75 minutes a week of vigorous aerobic exercise.

Moderate exercise includes: brisk walking, cycling, hiking, playing golf (when you carry your bag), slow team sport (basketball, volleyball), swimming, mowing the lawn.

Vigorous aerobic exercise includes: jogging or running, tennis, fast team sport (football, rugby), gym workouts (rowing or treadmill).

Walking

Walking is the easiest and cheapest way to keep fit. Recent research published in the US journal *Arteriosclerosis Thrombosis, and Vascular Biology* shows that walking is every bit as good for your heart as running and jogging. The British Heart Foundation advises that moderate-intensity aerobic exercise is the most effective type of activity for maintaining a healthy heart. Aerobic activity is any repetitive rhythmic exercise involving large muscle groups, such as legs, shoulders and arms.

Walking 'briskly' lowers the risk of heart disease, high cholesterol, high blood pressure and diabetes more than the same amount of energy used through vigorous exercise. A half-hour brisk walk is the equivalent of one hour of running. Not only will brisk walking aid weight management, it also improves your physical health and your chances of living a longer life. In time, bone strength will improve, as will balance and coordination. Further benefits include: improved mental health, reduced feelings of depression, clearer thinking, an elevated mood and a greater sense of self-esteem.

A person of average weight can expect to use around 350–400 calories per hour spent walking briskly. If you spend 150 minutes per week in brisk walking you can expect to use up to 1,000 calories.

'Brisk walking' means walking purposefully while swinging your arms and torso. For maximum effect and weight-loss maintenance, as you walk contract your stomach muscles, holding your buttocks tightly together.

Start slowly. Walk out of your home or place of work, keep going for five minutes, turn around and return. Do this for two to three days, then raise the time to 10 minutes, 15 minutes, 20 minutes. As you do this, build up to a speed of around 6 km (4 miles) per hour. As you become more used to brisk walking, stride out as if you are on a mission, or late for an appointment. You are not running, but almost. A useful test of your speed and effort is to try to sing. Can't do it? Great.

The only equipment you will need is a good pair of shoes to help absorb shock. A pedometer is handy for measuring your success in terms of distance walked and calories burnt. Several apps are available for showing your route and measuring distance walked, speed and paces taken, and calories burnt. Try MapMyWalk (Android devices) or RunKeeper (Apple devices). Alternatively, go to www.gmap-pedometer. com and use the site to either track your path, or help design walks of different distances, which you can print and keep for reference.

Running

When we exercise, using more calories than we take in through food, our fat stores are gradually used up. This means that fat from all over the body is lost. It is not possible to use specific exercises to isolate fat loss, such as belly or hip fat. Specific exercises will simply result in muscle development in the targeted areas.

Running has never been more popular, with marathons capturing the public imagination. Recreational running can be done by anyone, anywhere. All you need are suitable running shoes and clothing and you are away. A quick Google search will reveal any running clubs near where you live or work.

For many, the joy of running is that you can do it practically anywhere, without the need to join a club, or find a running track. Just head out of your front door and off you go.

If you have not run before, start out slowly. Alternate running and walking three or four times a week until you get used to running. Build up to around 5 km (3 miles) and try to run three to four times a week. You don't have to become a fanatic to gain results from running. Nor do you have to join a gym and slog away on a treadmill.

Pilates

Pilates is a fitness system that has been around for over 50 years. It is aimed at building muscle strength, flexibility, posture and balance. It demands complete concentration and as it employs a variety of apparatus, and is best learnt by attending an introductory Pilates class.

Yoga

Yoga dates back to the 15th century. It is not a religion; it is a holistic exercise activity widely used by athletes as part of their regular exercise regime. Recent research into the health benefits of yoga show that it outperformed aerobic exercises at improving balance, flexibility and physical strength. In hatha yoga, physical exercise is gained through posture, and is not only for the young, fit and flexible. Many practitioners are still enjoying yoga well into their eighties, claiming that they are more flexible, have improved posture and balance, sleep better and enjoy increased energy levels. As well as physical gains, yoga has a reputation for helping to develop a greater sense of well-being.

Yoga has also been shown to help reduce stress levels. Chronic stress leads to a consumption of foods high in sugar and fat and it is thought that regular yoga practice can help ward off obesity.

Tennis player Andy Murray credits his improved performance to his decision to practise yoga and believes that hatha yoga has transformed him both physically and mentally. Hatha yoga classes teach a variety of poses, which can form the core of a basic routine workout. If you want to get fit and stay fit, both physically and mentally, then yoga could be the regime for you. There will be plenty of classes to seek out near where you live.

Zumba Fitness

The Latin-inspired dance offers the opportunity to have fun, exercise and lose weight while dancing freely to up-tempo tracks. Zumba is a full body instructor-led improvised workout that has gained a huge following in recent years. It is particularly recommended as helping to develop a good cardiovascular respiratory system and improving your oxygen intake. Although not designed as a weight-loss regime, some studies suggest that a regular attendee may expect to use an incredible 500–750 calories in a well-instructed one-hour session.

Boot Camp

Based on the popularity of outdoor fitness training in the US, so-called boot camps are springing up everywhere in the UK and are well worth investigating if your schedule allows an early-morning start (around 6.30am). Run by qualified personal trainers, a typical boot camp operates in all weathers and may offer a range of high-energy activities ranging from boxing to running and circuit training, with all abilities and fitness levels catered for.

Usually open to anyone over 16, boot camps may typically last for four weeks and meet three times a week. Trainers are insured and ensure that there are no medical issues that might prohibit you from high-energy exercise.

SELF-MONITOR YOUR HEALTH AND FITNESS

Use self-monitoring to alter your health and fitness in a fundamental way by changing your habits and behaviour. Your body is very responsive – to the food you choose, the portions you take, the liquids you drink, the exercise you take and your sleep patterns.

Monitor your weight daily, at the same time, wearing the same clothes. The best time to check your weight is in the morning, after your shower, naked. Many diet regimes suggest that weekly weight checks are sufficient; we don't agree. A weekly check is highly dependent on what you ate and drank the day before, the regularity of your bowel movements, your water retention and your sleep patterns. By weighing yourself daily, any unusual weight blips (up or down) will be ironed out as your weekly weight pattern emerges. And don't worry if you suddenly put on 0.9 kg (2 lb) overnight. To gain a pound in actual weight you will need to have consumed a massive 3,500 calories over your recommended daily maximum in 24 hours. Unless you have overindulged, the curve on your daily weight chart should maintain its steady downward path.

There are numerous apps available that allow us to learn things about ourselves and help guide us towards changing our behaviour for the better. Here are some examples of the better apps. (This is by no means an exhaustive list; new and improved apps become available almost every day.)

HEALTH, FITNESS AND MENTAL AGILITY APPS

MyFitnessPal: a diet and fitness community, which provides the user with the tools and support needed to achieve personal weight-loss goals. 'We believe – and medical studies prove – that the best way to lose weight and keep it off forever is to simply keep track of the foods you eat. Gimmicky machines and fad diets don't work, so we designed a free website and mobile apps that make calorie counting and food tracking easy.'

Moves: automatically records any walking, cycling and running you do. You can view the distance, duration, steps and calories burnt for each activity. The app is always on, so there's no need to start and stop it. Just keep your phone in your pocket or your bag.

Endomondo: one of the highest-rated apps of its kind on Android and ideal for running, cycling, walking and any other distance-based activity.

- Track any outdoor sport including duration, distance, speed and calories burnt.
- Enter a workout manually, e.g. a treadmill run or weight training.
- Get audio feedback for every mile or kilometre while exercising.
- Get live pep talks from friends – they write a short text on the Endomondo website which is then read out to you seconds later.
- Set a distance goal and track your route on a map.
- Track your heart rate.
- View the history of your workouts and study split times per mile or kilometre.
- Sync workouts across multiple platforms.
- Post your workouts to your Facebook Timeline.
- See your friends' latest workouts in real time.

Sleep Cycle: a best-selling app that turns your mobile phone into a sleep-tracking device. Take it to bed and it will monitor your body movements throughout the night. As you approach wakefulness, Sleep Cycle assists you back to consciousness by playing gentle, soothing music. Your nightly sleep patterns are recorded in the form of a graph. By associating the readouts with the food, drink, exercise and behaviours of the previous evening, these can help you make changes which will give you more restful sleep and, it is claimed, can make you less anxious and depression prone.

Luminosity: offers exercises that help improve brain performance. Regular use improves memory, alertness, problem solving and flexibility. Luminosity has over 40 million users and the world's largest database on human cognition, which in turn is used to develop further the Luminosity cognitive training programme.

CHAPTER 15

MEDITATION AND SPIRITUAL WELL-BEING

What lies behind us and what lies before us are tiny matters compared to what lies within us.

Oliver Wendell Holmes

The monks' remarkably healthy and long lives must be at least partly due to their quiet, contemplative lifestyle, which carries with it few existential worries. Monks don't meditate as such, although they spend a good part of every day alone in their cells praying. As Father C. puts it: 'Even though we devote some time alone to our prayers, we are in fact praying continuously.' What he meant by this was that the monks mentally repeat the so-called 'Jesus prayer' over and over to themselves. This simple 12-word mantra is not oral; it is a prayer of the mind, repeated probably a thousand times a day, during work, at meals, even mentally during verbal conversations with others.

For some readers 'meditation' may suggest hours of staring into space, withdrawing from the world or chanting mystical mantras. You will forgiven for asking: 'How can 20 minutes of daily navel-gazing possibly do me any good?' However, the mind is an enormously powerful and underused human resource. No matter what religious beliefs you may or may not hold meditation can achieve fast and measurable results. Meditation has at times received a rather colourful press – many will recall the Beatles' flirtation with Transcendental Meditation during their collective search for enlightenment in the 1960s. Although they were only with the Maharishi Mahesh Yogi for a very short while, his teachings did have a marked influence on their lives and music; we would not have the 'White Album' without it and daily meditation helped John Lennon come off drugs completely.

In the 21st century, meditation has gained wider public acceptance. Many politicians, business leaders, actors, athletes and sports people acknowledge their debt to meditation. Just prior to his 2013 Wimbledon semi-final match, Novak Djokovic was seen meditating for an hour at the Buddhapadipa complex, a 10-minute walk away from the All England Club. Here was a tennis player who, as a younger athlete, seemed to have little control over his emotions, but since taking up meditation and yoga, all that has changed. Like many sports stars, Djokovic recognises that mental strength is every bit as important as physical strength and stamina.

SO – HOW CAN MEDITATION HELP YOU?

Meditation takes many forms. It is not restricted to religious purposes: it is found in many of today's secular contexts, counselling and psychotherapy in particular.

Findings from recent research studies have supported the view that regular meditation is linked to a variety of health benefits. These include reductions in:

- stress levels
- high blood pressure
- depression
- pain levels
- heart rate
- headaches

In addition, studies suggest that meditation can help to:

- develop your self-awareness
- clear your thinking
- give your life clarity and focus
- release you from a 'stuck state'
- improve your memory
- increase your attention span
- improve your empathy for others
- boost your self-esteem
- increase your reaction time
- improve your concentration
- accelerate your academic performance
- help you to relax

HOW TO MEDITATE

Meditation is not an innate skill. No one is born knowing how to meditate. We all know how to run – but to run a marathon we need training. And so it is with meditation. Peace of mind, resilience and emotional balance are not normal states for the majority of human beings. To achieve these desirable states of mind, we need training. Meditation techniques can be learnt quickly, but are no easy remedy and take discipline to master.

However, many newcomers to meditation find immediate benefits. Just taking time out to sit calmly and quietly for 20 minutes can offer a remarkable payback.

A 'normal' state of mind, though, does not mean an optimal state. The scope for development and improvement is vast and well within the grasp of most of us.

Meditation is not about achieving ecstatic states. Instead, it offers us the opportunity to examine the difference between outer and inner conditions to happiness. For example, how is it perfectly possible to be miserable when everything around us is sunny? We can observe our inner state – and all of us possess the potential to change and improve that state.

Sadness, negativity, jealousy, anger and irritation are all mental constructs of our own making. We can allow ourselves to wallow in them, or make a decision never to again. It's that simple. True mastery of the mind is freedom of the mind. As Father J. puts it: 'Conflict? Monks don't all think or act alike, so there can be conflict, yes, but we don't dwell on it. One hour later, and it's vanished.'

AN INTRODUCTORY LESSON

Set aside 20 minutes of your time when you can be alone. Turn off all possible means of distraction: mobiles, landlines, radio and television.

- Sit comfortably. Sit upright.
- Start by concentrating on your breathing. As you do so, become aware of the air going into and out of your nostrils. Pause and notice how it feels.

- How does your breathing affect the rest of your body? The movement of your chest and stomach? The rise and fall of your shoulders?
- Now become aware of the temperature: yours and that of the room itself.
- Listen for a while to any ambient sounds.
- Now that you are aware of your breathing and what's going on around you, take in these sensations. There is no need to analyse or explain them, just enjoy being curious about them, get to know them. You have now taken your mind to a subconscious level. Other thoughts of family, work and money begin to recede.
- Now concentrate on a positive state which you have previously experienced, for example that of unconditional love. Recall how you felt or feel when in that state. You may want to recall the place, or the people who shared this with you. Hold the memory there, in your mind's eye. Savour it for long enough to recall it at will.

If you continue to follow this path for 20 minutes a time over a few days, the very thought of 'unconditional love' will leap immediately into your mind. Congratulations – you have created another world for yourself.

DEALING WITH NEGATIVE EMOTIONS

Meditating can help us deal better with negative emotions. Negative emotions arise from negative thoughts. Thoughts have a life cycle: they spring into our head, linger for as long as we let them, and then, eventually, evaporate. We are always in control of the amount of time we allow thoughts to hover in our mind.

Think of a recurring negative emotion that you would like to banish. Stand back and, with your mind's eye, become aware of the emotion. Awareness is not the emotion itself. Do not try to suppress the emotion, simply concentrate on it. Now, get rid of it. Banish it. Now, bring it back and abandon it once more. By doing this continuously you build up the capacity to deal with the emotion when it first arrives and avoid being overwhelmed by it.

AFFIRMATION

Meditation is a great tool for reinforcing or affirming positive thoughts. Emile Coué, the father of conscious auto-suggestion, coined the well-known phrase: 'Every day, in every way, I am getting better and better.' He taught that internal conflict occurs between the will and the imagination, but the imagination is always stronger.

While meditating repeat to yourself your positive thought over and over, every day, at least 20 times, always in the same tone.

Some examples of affirming thoughts may include:

- I am no longer worried
- I feel better
- Now I can cope
- I have put that behind me
- Nothing can stop me from …

... AND FINALLY

The French psychoanalyst Charles Baudouin said: 'People are inclined to disbelieve the efficacy of anything simple.' This is particularly true of meditation. We vastly underestimate the power of the mind. Not everything has to be difficult to be of value. You will find as you progress with meditating that the process becomes easier and more natural. It can work wonders for your mind, body and spirit. Meditation will give you all the resources you need and will put you back in charge of your emotions. It will help you develop qualities that lie within you and build inner strength.

There are so many ways you can meditate and plenty of sources from which to gain more information and help. Good luck on your journey.

CHAPTER 16

MAINTAINING THE DIET

You have reached your goal weight – congratulations! Depending on how much you wanted to lose, it might have taken you a short time or a bit longer, but with perseverance and determination you have achieved your target.

Now what? It's a well-known cliché that keeping weight off is harder than losing it, so how do you stay at your target weight with the Mount Athos Diet?

Find what works for you – the beauty of the Mount Athos Diet is its variety. You know that you can balance your Feast Days with your Fast Days and still lose weight, and the same is true when it comes to maintaining your ideal weight. It may take a bit of juggling to discover what works for you, but you will come to realise what works and what doesn't. For example, you might stick to the Monday, Wednesday and Friday Fast Day pattern, replacing Sunday's Moderation Day with a second Feast Day. Or, you might stick to just one Feast Day, and six Moderation Days. For some, the Fast Days provide a natural break and allow for a pause during the week, but you might choose to shift the ratio of Fast Days to Moderation Days to 2:4 rather than 3:3 (meaning 2 Fast Days and

4 Moderation Days per week). For some, it may be that the Mount Athos Diet without any modifications is what will keep you at your goal weight – dependent on so many personal factors (height, activity levels, age, etc.), your body may have reached a natural equilibrium – so keep doing what you have done so far.

Experiment – the best approach is to make gradual increases and monitor the effect this has on your weight. Give yourself a couple of weeks of experimenting, monitor closely, and assess how this affects your weight. If you don't gain any weight, try another fortnight of experimentation, and monitor again. Bear in mind that one of the core values of the Mount Athos Diet is to eat when you are hungry and stop when you are full. One of the reasons calorie counting can be problematic is that it deals in numerical allowances leading dieters to eat the maximum amount of food they can have, and doesn't teach you to listen to your body. Also, calorie counting works with a set limit that doesn't vary day by day. Naturally, the body may be hungrier on some days and less hungry other times. This natural variation may fluctuate daily, weekly or seasonally. Above all, listen to your body and try to work Fast Days, Moderation Days and Feast Days around the times you are naturally most and least hungry. That way, you are working with your body, not battling against your natural impulses.

Maintain a routine – whatever you decide, it's important to stick to the good habits you learnt with the Mount Athos Diet. Try to identify the specific habits you found easiest and stick to them – if you are already doing this, it means that you are halfway there. Keep up with your exercise – this is very important as your current metabolism is likely to have been accelerated by your exercise plan. Limit the days on which you drink alcohol. Keep snacking to a minimum. Plan ahead. Earlier in the book we suggested getting out your calendar and planning your Feast Days, which is a strategy that could be useful well into the maintenance phase of the diet. You are looking to find ways to avoid slipping back to your old habits.

Be realistic – it's easy to believe that your body has changed in more ways than the weight loss. Don't suddenly decide you can eat whatever you fancy. If you have previously been the type of person who gains weight easily, this is unlikely to be different now. The older we get, the slower our metabolism becomes, meaning that what you might once have eaten regularly a decade ago without gaining weight may not be the case now.

Monitor your weight – set a limit of a few kilos or pounds above your ideal weight, for example 1.3–2.3 kg (3–5 lb) and keep checking your progress. Once you reach that limit, take action. It's easier to tackle a few kilos or pounds gained after a particularly indulgent week, for example, than it is to bury your head in the sand and pretend it's not happening, and risk much greater weight gain a few weeks down the line, which may feel insurmountable.

Take action – don't put off tackling a few kilos' or pounds' weight gain. Set yourself a target, much as you did when you began the Mount Athos Diet, and look forward to reaching it. Another action you may need to take is to routinely patrol your kitchen storecupboards to ensure that you continue to remove temptation. Don't shop when you are hungry. Beware of portion sizes increasing.

Be kind to yourself – many people beat themselves up about weight gain, which isn't productive. Instead, accept that you may have indulged a little too often, and use the knowledge, understanding and skills you have learnt on the Mount Athos Diet to tackle the situation. And ask friends and family to support you in the way in which they did while you were losing weight. It's much easier to find ways to tackle weight gain when you feel happy and supported.

Remember that one indulgent meal won't undo all that hard work and will not make you gain back the weight you lost; the reason we gain or lose weight is through consistent eating habits across days, weeks and months. This is true of weight loss AND of weight gain. It's all about the balance, and the Mount Athos Diet is the perfect way to ensure you learn a new balance in your life. It may take some time to reach the right equilibrium for you, but you will get there. It's worth putting in the effort as this is what will help you to maintain your ideal weight for months and years to come.

CHAPTER 17

FAST DAY RECIPES

BREAKFASTS

Stewed Apple with Oats

Serves 1

1 medium Bramley apple
1 tsp ground cinnamon or mixed spice, to taste
2 tbsp porridge (rolled) oats
1 tsp maple syrup or honey, to taste

Peel and slice the apple, and place in a saucepan. Add the cinnamon or mixed spice and a splash of water. Bring to a simmer over a medium heat, then stir and cover. Every so often, check, stir and use a wooden spoon to break up the apple pieces as they soften. This will take about 10–15 minutes. When the apple is soft, place in a bowl and add the oats. Stir to combine, then top with the maple syrup or honey.

Notes:
- Add a dollop of Greek yogurt on Moderation Days.
- You can also cook this in the microwave in a bowl with a lid for about 5 minutes on full power. Be sure to stir and mash once or twice during cooking.

Grilled Peaches
Serves 1

1 peach
1 tsp maple syrup or honey
1 tsp ground cinnamon or mixed spice, to taste

Preheat the grill to medium.

Halve the peach and remove the stone. Place, cut side up, on a baking tray or dish. Mix the syrup or honey with the spice, then brush on to the cut side of each peach. Place under the grill for 5 minutes, until the top has browned and the fruit has begun to soften. Serve on its own or with Porridge (see page 136).

Notes:
- Serve with Greek yogurt on Moderation Days.
- This recipe is also delicious with plums.

Banana Toast
Serves 1

1 slice wholegrain bread (no butter)
½–1 ripe banana
honey, maple syrup or ground cinnamon, to taste (optional)

Toast the bread. Slice the banana and gently mash down on to the bread. Top with a drizzle of honey, maple syrup or cinnamon.

Porridge
Serves 1

50 g (1¾ oz) porridge (rolled) oats
pinch of salt
1 tsp honey (optional)

Put the oats, 250 ml (9 fl oz) water and salt into a saucepan over a low heat. Stir gently while the water heats through and the porridge thickens slowly, at least 5 minutes. Stirring well will ensure a smooth and creamy consistency. When cooked, add the honey if liked or top with fresh fruit.

Note:
- Adjust the quantity of water depending on how thick or otherwise you like your porridge.

Full Greek Breakfast
Serves 2

400 g (14 oz) can baked beans
2 medium tomatoes
4–6 medium portabella or brown mushrooms, cleaned
   with damp kitchen paper and patted dry
olive oil spray
salt and freshly ground black pepper
small handful of fresh parsley, finely chopped

Preheat the grill to medium.

Heat the beans in a saucepan. Halve the tomatoes and cut the mushrooms into thick 1-cm (½-in) slices, trimming the stalks if necessary. Spray the mushrooms with a little olive oil, season lightly with salt and pepper and place on a baking sheet. Put the sheet on the highest shelf in the oven, beneath the grill and cook for about 10 minutes, turning occasionally until done. Alternatively, preheat the oven to 200°C/400°F/ Gas mark 6, cover the mushrooms with foil and place on the top shelf of the oven.

Sprinkle the tomatoes and mushrooms with the parsley and serve with the beans.

Grilled Grapefruit
Serves 1

1 grapefruit
½ tsp honey or maple syrup for drizzling
¼–½ tsp mixed spice, to taste (optional)

Preheat the grill to medium.

Cut the grapefruit in half along its equator and place on a baking tray or dish. Drizzle a little honey or maple syrup over the top and sprinkle with spice, if liked. Grill for 5 minutes then serve.

Note:
- This is a very light breakfast. Team with a slice of toast and sugar-free fruit jam for a more substantial meal.

Muesli with Fruit Juice
Serves 1

Home-made muesli:
*a mix of porridge (rolled) oats, wheat flakes, wheat
    germ, pumpkin and sunflower seeds, walnuts, pecan
    nuts and hazelnuts, roughly chopped, toasted flaked
    almonds, raisins and dried blueberries*

To serve:
*¼ sharp apple, such as Cox's or Granny Smith
cloudy apple juice, to taste
½ tsp maple syrup or honey*

To make home-made muesli: combine all the muesli ingredients together in a container.

Place 4–5 dessertspoons of muesli into a bowl, then grate over the apple and pour over the juice to taste. For added sweetness, add a very small amount of maple syrup or honey.

Note:
• Home-made muesli is far nicer and much more satisfying than most of the shop-bought varieties. It also allows you to retain control over unwanted ingredients, such as added sugar and salt. Just mix your preferred quantities of muesli ingredients together and keep in an airtight container.

SALADS

Hearty Harissa Salad
Serves 2

½ medium butternut squash, peeled and deseeded
1 tbsp harissa paste
olive oil spray
400 g(14 oz) can chickpeas, drained and rinsed
250 g (9 oz) asparagus
1 red pepper, sliced
100 g (3½ oz) salad leaves
juice of ½ lemon
salt and freshly ground black pepper

Preheat the oven to 180°C/350°F/Gas mark 4.

Cube the butternut squash into 1–2-cm (½–¾-in) dice. Mix the harissa and 1 tbsp water together in a bowl, then add the diced squash and stir to coat thoroughly. Line a baking tray with baking parchment, then spray with oil spray. Remove the squash from the bowl with a slotted spoon and add to the lined tray. Roast in the oven for about 20–30 minutes. Add the chickpeas to the bowl with any remaining harissa mixture. Tumble together, then tip into another roasting tin and roast in the oven for 20 minutes, or until the chickpeas have shrunk and become crunchy.

Meanwhile, spray a griddle or stovetop grill pan with oil spray and place over the heat. When hot, place the asparagus and pepper slices in the pan. Keep an eye on them and turn the vegetables frequently, giving them an even coating of charred stripes. Check the asparagus is cooked by testing the stems with the tip of a sharp knife – it should slide in easily. Divide the salad leaves between 2 plates, top with the squash, chickpeas, asparagus and pepper. Pour over the lemon juice and add salt and pepper to taste.

Note:
Optional dressing for Moderation Days:

250 g (9 oz) Greek yogurt
1 garlic clove, peeled and crushed
5 cm (2 in) cucumber, peeled and finely diced
salt and freshly ground black pepper

For the dressing, mix the ingredients together and add salt and pepper to taste. Ideally, leave for 30 minutes or so to allow the flavours to develop (so make this first). Serve alongside the salad, 1–2 tbsp per person.

Roast Pepper, Spinach and Orange Salad

Serves 2 as a main course or 4 as a side dish

> *2 red or orange peppers*
> *1 large orange*
> *250 g (9 oz) spinach, washed*
> *2 tbsp pine nuts*
> *1 tbsp balsamic vinegar*
> *salt and freshly ground black pepper*

Preheat the grill to high.

Halve the peppers, place them on a baking tray and put under the grill.

Meanwhile, cut the top and bottom off the orange, then slice away the orange peel and pith. Slice down the membranes of each orange segment leaving individual pieces of fruit. Put the spinach and orange together into a bowl. When all slices of the orange have been sliced away, squeeze the remaining pith and membranes to release the juice into a separate bowl.

When the pepper skins are blackened, place in a plastic bag and close to contain the steam. After a few minutes, remove a pepper from the bag (leaving the rest sealed) and carefully remove the skin, stalk and membrane. Slice the flesh into bite-sized chunks and add to the bowl with the spinach and orange. Repeat for the remaining peppers.

Toast the pine nuts in a dry pan until they begin to colour and smell nutty. Set aside.

Add the vinegar to the orange juice and season with salt and pepper to taste. Pour the dressing over the salad, top with the pine nuts and serve.

Mount Athos White Bean Salad
Serves 6

2 x 400 g (14 oz) cans of butter beans, drained and
*   rinsed*
10 spring onions
handful of fresh flat-leaf parsley
2 tsp oregano leaves (preferably fresh)
juice of ½ lemon
1 tbsp olive oil
salt and freshly ground black pepper

Put the butter beans in a large bowl. Chop the spring onions
and parsley and add to the butter beans, along with the
oregano, lemon juice, olive oil and seasoning. Mix well and
add more lemon juice and seasoning if liked.

Serve warm.

Indian Salad

Adjust quantities to suit:
red cabbage, cucumber, grated carrot, spring onion,
    mango, grated coconut (preferably fresh but dry will
    do), pomegranate seeds, coriander, pumpkin seeds
fresh lime juice, to serve

Finely chop all the vegetables and mix together in a large bowl. Serve with fresh lime juice.

SOUPS

Moroccan Carrot and Chickpea Soup
Serves 2

olive oil spray
1 celery stick, trimmed and finely chopped
2 medium carrots, peeled and finely chopped
1 medium onion, peeled and finely chopped
1 garlic clove, peeled and crushed
2 tsp ground cumin
400 g (14 oz) can chopped tomatoes
400 ml (14 fl oz) vegetable stock (see page 186 or use a
*   good alternative such as Marigold bouillon powder)*
1 tsp sugar
½ can (220 g/7 oz) chickpeas
juice of ½ lemon
large handful of fresh coriander leaves, chopped
chilli powder, for sprinkling (optional)

Lightly baste a non-stick pan with a fine spray of olive oil, then add the celery, carrots, onion and garlic to the pan and set over a low heat. Stir, cover with a lid and steam-fry for 10 minutes or until the vegetables are softened. Add the cumin, then stir and cook for 2 minutes. Add the tomatoes, stock and sugar, then bring to the boil. Reduce the heat and simmer gently for 5 minutes. Add the chickpeas, lemon juice and coriander and heat through until hot.

Blitz the mixture with a hand-held blender until about half the soup is puréed. If you like it hot, sprinkle with chilli powder.

Note:
• Serve with lightly toasted mini pitta breads.

Tuscan Bean Soup
Serves 4

1 large onion, peeled
2 small carrots, peeled and trimmed
2 celery sticks, trimmed
2 garlic cloves, peeled
large handful of fresh parsley
olive oil spray
400 g (14 oz) carton passata
1 tbsp tomato purée
1 red chilli
1 litre (1¾ pints) vegetable stock (see page 186)
400 g (14 oz) can borlotti beans, drained
1 red pepper, cut into 2-cm (¾-in) square pieces
2 medium courgettes, cut into 2-cm (¾-in) pieces
salt and freshly ground black pepper

In a food processor, whizz up the first 5 ingredients until you have finely chopped vegetables.

Spray a few squirts of olive oil spray into a heavy-based pan and set over a low heat. When hot, add the finely chopped vegetables and cook gently, stirring frequently for 20–30 minutes until the vegetables are stewed and softened.

Add the passata, tomato purée, chilli and stock and bring to the boil. Reduce the heat and simmer for about 30 minutes or until the soup has thickened and reduced. Add the borlotti beans, red pepper and courgettes and cook for a further 15 minutes. Remove the chilli, check for seasoning and serve.

Note:
• Moderation Day: add a few shavings of Parmesan to serve, and a small chunk of crusty bread.

Herby Vegetable Soup
Serves 4

olive oil spray
2 medium onions, peeled and roughly chopped
2 celery sticks, trimmed and chopped
1 medium leek, trimmed and chopped
1 tsp fresh thyme leaves
2 medium carrots, peeled and chopped
2 medium potatoes, peeled and chopped into 2.5-cm
  (1-in) pieces
½ medium butternut squash, peeled and chopped
1 litre (1¾ pints) vegetable stock (see page 186 or use a
  good alternative such as Marigold bouillon powder)
1 generous stem of freshly picked rosemary, finely
  chopped
salt and freshly ground black pepper

Spray a few squirts of olive oil spray into a large pan and set over a medium heat. When hot, add the onions, celery, leek and thyme and stir, adding a small amount of water if it begins to stick to the base. Cover with a lid and steam-fry for 10 minutes, or until the vegetables have softened. Add the carrots, potatoes and squash, stir, then pour in the stock. Increase the heat until you get a gentle boil going, then add the rosemary to taste. Allow the soup to simmer away quietly for 30 minutes or so, or until the vegetables are tender. It is up to you how firm you like your vegetables and, indeed, whether you choose to whizz it up in a blender, mash it or leave it rustic. Taste for seasoning, and add more salt if it needs it and a few grinds of black pepper.

Carrot and Cumin Soup
Serves 2

  olive oil spray
  1 medium onion, peeled and chopped
  ½ tsp ground cumin
  ½ tsp ground ginger
  400 g(14 oz) carrots, peeled and sliced
  850 ml (1½ pints) vegetable stock (see page 186 or use
    a good alternative such as Marigold bouillon powder)
  15 g (½ oz) dried soup pasta
  salt and freshly ground black pepper

Spray a few squirts of olive oil spray into a medium pan and heat over a medium heat. When hot, add the onion and stir-fry until the onion is beginning to go translucent and colour slightly. Add the spices and carrots, then pour in the stock. Cover with a lid and simmer for 20 minutes, or until the carrots are soft. Mash, blend or whizz in a food processor, then return the soup to the rinsed-out pan. Add the pasta and seasoning to taste and cook for a further 5 minutes until the pasta is cooked through. Serve.

Japanese Noodle Soup
Serves 1

> *about 500 ml/18 fl oz per person vegetable stock (see*
> *page 186 or use a good alternative such as Marigold*
> *bouillon powder)*
> *1 garlic clove, peeled and crushed*
> *1-cm (½-in) piece of fresh ginger, peeled and crushed*
> *1 dried chilli or ¼ tsp chilli flakes*
> *1 tbsp mirin (Japanese rice wine)*
> *splash of sesame oil*
> *2 tbsp soy sauce*
> *mangetout, chopped mushrooms, peas, shredded Savoy*
> *cabbage*
> *90 g (3¼ oz) wholewheat or buckwheat (soba) noodles*
> *chopped spring onions and torn fresh coriander leaves,*
> *to serve*

Make up the soup base by combining the stock, garlic, ginger, chilli, mirin, sesame oil and soy sauce in a medium saucepan and bring to a simmer. Add the vegetables in the order in which they will cook (i.e. mangetout first, cabbage last).

In a separate pan, boil enough water to cover the noodles, then add the noodles and cook until just soft, then drain. Once the soup and vegetables are cooked, add the drained noodles and top with spring onions and coriander. Serve immediately.

Note:
- This is an endlessly adaptable recipe. Scale it up according to how many mouths you have to feed, or adjust the vegetable components to suit what's in your fridge.

Pea Soup
Serves 4–6

> *olive oil spray*
> *1 garlic clove, peeled and chopped*
> *1 medium leek, white part only, trimmed and chopped*
> *2 large shallots, peeled and chopped*
> *1 medium potato, diced small (optional – the recipe*
> *works equally well without)*
> *1 litre (1¾ pints) vegetable stock (see page 186 or use a*
> *good alternative such as Marigold bouillon powder)*
> *500 g (1 lb 2 oz) frozen or fresh peas*
> *small bunch of fresh mint, roughly chopped*
> *salt and ground white pepper*

Spray a large pan with a few squirts of olive oil. Add the garlic, leek and shallots, cover with a lid and steam-fry them over a low heat until softened. Add the potato and stock and simmer until the potato is tender. Add the peas and mint and cook until the peas are tender. Purée, adding more stock if necessary to adjust the consistency. Check the seasoning, adding salt and white pepper to taste.

Note:
- On a Moderation Day, you could add 1 tbsp Greek yogurt to serve.

Turkish Spiced Chickpea Soup
Serves 4

olive oil spray
1 medium red onion, peeled and thinly sliced
15 g (½ oz) finely chopped fresh ginger
240 g (9 oz) canned chickpeas
500 ml (18 fl oz) vegetable stock (see page 186 or use a
*   good alternative such as Marigold bouillon powder)*
250 g (9 oz) watercress, washed
150 g (5 oz) spinach leaves, washed
2 tsp granulated sugar
sea salt and freshly ground black pepper
1 tsp rosewater
3 medium or 2 large carrots, peeled and chopped into
*   2-cm (¾-in) dice*
3 tsp ras el hanout
½ tsp ground cinnamon

Preheat the oven to 220°C/425°F/Gas mark 7.

Spray a few squirts of olive oil spray into a heavy-based pan, add the onion and ginger and cook gently until soft, translucent and a pale gold colour. Add half the chickpeas, stock, watercress, spinach, sugar and a small pinch of salt. Bring to a rolling boil and cook for no more than 2 minutes, just to wilt the leaves. Leave to cool before blending into a smooth soup. Add the rosewater and check the seasoning.

Line a large baking dish with baking parchment. Put the carrots into a bowl. Add the ras el hanout, cinnamon and 1 tsp sea salt and spread over the base of the baking dish. Bake in the oven for 15 minutes then add the remaining chickpeas.

Stir well and cook for a further 10 minutes. Check that the carrots still have some bite; do not overcook. Set aside.

Reheat the soup and the roasted carrots and chickpeas if necessary. Pour the soup into 4 bowls and add the roasted carrots and chickpeas.

Note:
• Top with Greek yogurt on a Moderation Day.

Mount Athos Vegetable Soup
Serves 6

250 g (9 oz) carrots, peeled
500 g (1 lb 2 oz) waxy potatoes, peeled
3 celery sticks, trimmed
1 large onion, peeled
1 medium leek, trimmed
2 red peppers, cored
1 medium bunch of fresh parsley
1 medium bunch of fresh dill
1 tsp ground cumin
salt and freshly ground black pepper
juice of 2 lemons

Chop all the vegetables, ensuring you have chunks of roughly the same size. Finely chop the herbs. Bring 3 litres (5 pints) water to the boil in a large pan. Add the vegetables and cook for 5 minutes, then stir and add the parsley, dill and cumin. Reduce the heat and cook for about 20 minutes, but make sure you test the vegetables frequently; they should retain some 'bite'. Season with salt and pepper to taste, then add the lemon juice.

Mount Athos Lentil Soup
Serves 4

400 g (14 oz) can plum tomatoes
1 small onion, peeled and grated
2 garlic cloves, peeled and sliced
½ tsp granulated sugar
2 bay leaves
salt and freshly ground black pepper
400 g (14 oz) can green lentils, drained
1 tbsp red wine vinegar
½ tsp dried oregano or handful of fresh oregano,
*   chopped*

Blend the tomatoes and their juice until you have a smooth paste. In a large pan, cook the onion and garlic in 6 tbsp water until soft and the water has evaporated. Pour in 750 ml (1¼ pints) water, then add the tomato paste, sugar, bay leaves and salt and pepper. Bring to the boil and cook for 10–15 minutes. Add the canned lentils, vinegar and oregano and heat until piping hot. Check for seasoning and add salt, pepper, extra oregano or vinegar, if necessary. Remove the bay leaves before serving.

Note:
• Serve with olives on the side.

Mount Athos Bean Soup
Serves 6

1 large onion, peeled and grated
2 large carrots, peeled and sliced
1 celery stick, peeled and chopped
1 small dried red chilli
1 large green pepper, deseeded and chopped
400 g (14 oz) can tomatoes
1 tsp granulated sugar
1 tbsp red wine vinegar
4 tbsp finely chopped fresh parsley
400 g (14 oz) can pinto or red kidney beans
400 g (14 oz) can white beans
salt and freshly ground black pepper

Put the onion in a large pan with 120 ml (4 fl oz) water and cook over a medium heat, stirring until softened and the water has evaporated. Add the carrots, celery, dried red chilli and green pepper and cook for about 10 minutes until softened. Stir in the tomatoes, sugar, vinegar, parsley, beans, salt and pepper and 500 ml (18 fl oz) hot water. Cover with a lid and simmer gently for 30 minutes. When thickened, the soup is ready (add extra water should you need to).

Note:
• Serve with olives on the side.

Butternut Squash Soup
Serves 6

1 large butternut squash, peeled and chopped into
   2.5-cm (1-in) cubes
1 tsp olive oil
1 tsp chilli flakes
1 tsp cumin seeds
salt and freshly ground black pepper
1 medium white onion, peeled and diced
2 medium carrots, peeled and roughly diced
3 garlic cloves, peeled and minced
1 fresh rosemary sprig, leaves chopped
400 g (14 oz) can green lentils, drained
2 bay leaves
1.25 litres (2 pints) vegetable stock (see page 186 or
   use a good alternative such as Marigold bouillon
   powder), or water
1 tbsp wine vinegar

Preheat the oven to 200°C/400°F/Gas mark 6 and line a roasting tin with baking parchment.

Place the squash in a bowl with ½ tsp of the olive oil, then sprinkle with the chilli flakes, cumin seeds and a little salt and black pepper. Tip the squash mixture into the lined roasting tin and roast in the oven for 30–40 minutes, taking care not to burn the squash.

In a pan, gently sweat the onion, carrots, garlic and rosemary in the remaining olive oil for 10 minutes, until the onions are soft and translucent. Remove from the heat and add the lentils, bay leaves and stock or water. Return to the heat then add the roasted squash and cook gently for about 5 minutes. Adjust the seasoning and add the vinegar. Process two-thirds of the soup in a blender or food processor until silky and velvety. Reserve some chunks of butternut squash and blend the remaining soup lightly, making sure you retain some texture. Add the whole butternut squash pieces and pour in more water if the consistency is too thick, then serve.

Note:
- On Moderation Days serve each bowl with a spoonful of Greek yogurt added just before serving.

MAIN MEALS: SUBSTANTIAL STEWS, CURRIES, PASTA AND BAKES

Mediterranean Ragout
Serves 4

olive oil spray
2 small onions, peeled and cut into half moons
2 garlic cloves, peeled and chopped
1 celery stick, trimmed and chopped
½ tsp fennel seeds
½ tsp dried oregano
½ tsp dried thyme
1 red pepper, cored and cut into 2.5-cm (1-in) pieces
1 yellow pepper, cored and cut into 2.5-cm (1-in) pieces
½ medium courgette, trimmed and diced
1 medium sweet potato, cut into 2.5-cm (1-in) pieces
3 mushrooms, wiped and chopped
400 g (14 oz) can tomatoes
1 tbsp apple juice
400 g (14 oz) can black beans or chickpeas, drained
salt and freshly ground black pepper

Spray a few squirts of olive oil spray into a heavy-based pan and set over a medium heat. When hot, add the onions, garlic, celery and herbs and cook for 5 minutes or so, until softened. Add the remaining vegetables and cook, stirring frequently, until the vegetables are beginning to brown slightly. Add the tomatoes, then fill the can halfway up with water and pour into the pan. Finally, add the apple juice and the black beans or chickpeas. Reduce the heat to low–medium, so it's just bubbling gently and cook for 30 minutes, or until the ragout is thick and soupy. Season with salt and pepper and serve.

Note:
- Serve with jacket potatoes and plenty of green vegetables.

Spaghetti Arrabiatta

Serves 4

olive oil spray
1 medium onion, peeled and thinly sliced
2 garlic cloves, crushed, peeled and chopped
1 fresh chilli, deseeded and sliced (or use dried), or to taste
400 g (14 oz) can chopped tomatoes
400 g (14 oz) penne rigate, rigatoni or spaghetti
salt
small handful of fresh basil leaves, to serve

Spray a few squirts of olive oil spray into a pan large enough to hold the pasta and set over the heat. When hot, add the onion and cook gently for about 10 minutes. Add the garlic and cook for a further 5 minutes. Add the chilli and tomatoes and cook for a further 30 minutes, or until the sauce thickens and darkens in colour (if it becomes too thick, add a dash of cold water).

Meanwhile, bring a large pan of water to the boil, add the pasta and cook according to the instructions on the packet. Finally, taste the sauce, adding salt and more chilli, if needed, then add the cooked pasta to the sauce, stirring well. Cook for a further minute, then serve with basil leaves torn on the top.

Note:

- On Moderation Days, add a small amount of shaved or grated Parmesan to serve.

Moroccan Chickpea and Squash Stew
Serves 4–6

1 tsp ground ginger
1 tsp ground cumin
1 tsp ground paprika
¼ tsp turmeric
¼ tsp cayenne pepper
½ tsp ground cinnamon
olive oil spray
1 medium onion, peeled and cut into fine half rings
400 g (14 oz) can plum tomatoes
400 g (14 oz) can chickpeas, drained
300 g (11 oz) butternut squash (or other squash,
  pumpkin, etc.), peeled, deseeded and cut into 1-cm
  (½-in) dice (or larger if you like a stew with firmer
  veg and a slightly thinner sauce)
2 tbsp raisins
4 dried apricots, cut into 5-mm (¼-in) dice
500 ml (18 fl oz) vegetable stock (see page 186 or use a
  good alternative such as Marigold bouillon powder)
½ large courgette, trimmed and cut into 1-cm (½-in)
  dice
1 tbsp finely chopped fresh coriander
1 tbsp finely chopped fresh parsley

To serve:
couscous, bulgur wheat, quinoa or similar grain of your
  fancy
harissa paste

Combine the spices in a cup and set aside. Wipe the oil in the base of a large pan and set over a medium-high heat. When hot, add the onion and stir-fry for 3 minutes or so, until the onion has started to brown (add water if necessary to stop the onion burning). Add the spices from the cup, stir once, then add the tomatoes. Stir and cook for 3–4 minutes, or until the tomatoes have softened. Add the chickpeas, squash, raisins, apricots and stock and bring to a simmer. Cover with a lid, reduce the heat and cook for 15 minutes or so. The pan should be bubbling away nicely. When the squash is just tender when pierced with the point of a knife, add the courgette and simmer, uncovered, stirring occasionally, for a further 10 minutes, or until the courgette has softened to your liking. Add the coriander and parsley just before serving – give it a couple of minutes to cook down as parsley can be a bit on the tough side.

To serve, put a moderate mound of couscous or whatever you are having on each plate (around the size of one cupped hand). Make a well in the centre and put a chunky spoonful of stew in the well. Dampen the surrounding couscous generously with some of the sauce, and serve with harissa on the side.

Black Bean Chilli

Serves 4

olive oil spray
1 onion, peeled and finely chopped
3 garlic cloves, peeled and finely chopped
1 green pepper, cored and finely chopped
1 red chilli, finely chopped
1½ tsp ground cumin
2 tsp paprika
½ tsp dried thyme
½ tsp dried sage
1 tsp dried oregano
¼ tsp cayenne pepper
2 x 400 g (14 oz) cans black beans or other canned
  beans, drained
400 g (14 oz) can plum tomatoes
3 tbsp chopped fresh coriander leaves
½ tsp salt

To serve:
cooked brown rice
avocado slices

Spray a few squirts of olive oil spray into a large pan and set the pan over a medium heat. When hot, add the onion, garlic, green pepper and chilli and fry for 5 minutes, until just browned. Reduce the heat and continue to cook for a further 2 minutes, before adding the cumin, paprika, thyme, sage, oregano and cayenne. Stir and add the black beans, tomatoes, coriander and salt. Fill the tomato can with water and pour into the pan. Bring to the boil before covering with a lid. Reduce the heat to a gentle simmer and cook for 45 minutes. For the final 15 minutes, uncover and allow the sauce to thicken. Serve with brown rice and slices of avocado.

Notes:
- On Moderation Days, add a spoonful of Greek yogurt or a small amount of grated Cheddar to serve.
- This also works as a wrap filling so use any leftovers for lunch the next day.

Vegetable Tagine
Serves 4

olive oil spray
2 medium onions, peeled and roughly chopped into
    large chunks
2 garlic cloves, peeled and crushed
2 tsp paprika
3 tsp ground cumin
2 tsp ground coriander
pinch of saffron threads (or 1 tsp turmeric)
1 tsp ground ginger
3 medium carrots, peeled and chopped into 2.5-cm
    (1-in) chunks
4 medium potatoes or 1 medium sweet potato, peeled
    and cut into 2.5-cm (1-in) dice
350 g (12 oz) green beans, trimmed
1 red pepper, cored and sliced into 2.5-cm (1-in) pieces
½ lemon, cut into 2 quarters
400 g (14 oz) can chopped tomatoes
400 g (14 oz) can chickpeas, drained
small bunch each of fresh parsley and mint
1 tbsp chopped green olives
75 g (2½ oz) sultanas
salt and freshly ground black pepper
2 tsp harissa paste

Spray a few squirts of olive oil spray on the tagine base and
set over the heat. When hot, add the onions and cook gently
for 10 minutes or so, until soft and translucent. Add the garlic
and fry for 1 minute (make sure it does not burn), then add the

spices and cook for 3 minutes. Add all the remaining vege-tables, the lemon quarters, canned tomatoes and chickpeas and top up with enough water to barely cover the ingredi-ents. Cover with the tagine top and cook over a low heat for 30 minutes, testing the potatoes as you go. Finally, throw in all the herbs, olives and sultanas and cook for a further 10 minutes. Taste for seasoning, stir in the harissa and serve.

Note:

• This is delicious with couscous, rice or pitta bread.

Greek Baked Butter Beans

Serves 4

olive oil spray
1 medium onion, peeled and sliced into fine half rings
1 medium carrot, peeled and cut into thick slices
400 g (14 oz) can chopped tomatoes
400 g (14 oz) can butter beans, drained
2–3 tbsp finely chopped fresh parsley
1 tsp dried oregano
salt and freshly ground black pepper

Preheat the oven to 170°C/338°F/Gas mark 3.

Oil a heavy-based, ovenproof casserole dish and set over a medium heat. When hot, add the onion and carrot and stir-fry for 5 minutes. Add the tomatoes and cook for a further 10 minutes. Add the beans, parsley, oregano, salt and pepper to the casserole, together with 500 ml (18 fl oz) water. Stir, cover with a lid then cook in the oven for 2 hours.

Note:

- Serve with bread, salad and olives for a traditional, simple Greek meal.

Briam
Serves 4

4 large potatoes
olive oil spray
1 medium onion, peeled and diced
4 garlic cloves, peeled and finely minced
25 g (1 oz) fresh dill, chopped
small handful of fresh parsley, chopped
½ tsp dried oregano
4 fresh mint leaves
4 tbsp concentrated tomato paste
salt and freshly ground black pepper
4 large tomatoes, sliced
2 medium courgettes, trimmed and thinly sliced

Preheat the oven to 220°C/425°F/Gas mark 7. Peel and boil the potatoes until just tender. Drain and slice into 5-mm (¼-in) rounds then set aside.

Spray a few squirts of olive oil spray into a large pan and set the pan over the heat. When hot, add the onion and sauté gently until translucent. Add the garlic and sauté for 1 minute, then add the herbs, 1 tbsp of tomato paste and 150 ml (5 fl oz) water. Bring to the boil, cover with a lid, reduce the heat and simmer for about 15 minutes. Add more water if it starts to dry out.

Spread the onion mixture over the base of a baking dish, then layer half the potato slices on top and season lightly with salt and pepper. Layer the tomato slices on top of the potatoes. Season lightly. Next, add the remaining potatoes. Season lightly and add 1 tbsp tomato paste. Finally, add the courgette slices and top with the remaining 2 tbsp tomato paste. Cover with foil and bake for 1 hour, or until the vegetables have cooked through and are very tender, checking halfway through cooking and adding a little more water, if needed.

Lentil Dal
Serves 4

250 g (9 oz) red lentils
1 onion, peeled and cut into half moons
2 garlic cloves, peeled but left whole
2 bay leaves
½ tsp turmeric
1 fresh chilli
salt and freshly ground black pepper
rice, to serve

For the tarka:
¼ tsp asofoetida
¼ tsp ground fenugreek
½ tsp chilli flakes
1 tsp black mustard seeds
1 tsp cumin seeds
vegetable oil spray
2 garlic cloves, peeled and finely sliced
1 small tomato, finely chopped

Put the lentils, 900 ml (1½ pints) water, onion, garlic, bay leaves, turmeric and chilli into a large pan. Place over a medium heat, bring to the boil then leave, uncovered, to simmer for 20 minutes.

While the lentils are simmering, mix together the dry ingredients for the tarka in a small bowl or cup, and start cooking the rice to serve. When the lentils are cooked, remove the pan from the heat and remove the chilli and bay leaves with a slotted spoon. Use the back of a wooden spoon to break up the garlic cloves a little, then season with salt and pepper.

Brush the base of a small heavy-based saucepan with a small amount of vegetable oil, then add 1 tbsp water and set over the heat. When hot, add the garlic slices and allow to sizzle, but make sure they don't burn as this will make the garlic taste bitter. Throw in the dry spices, and fry until they begin to crackle and pop. When the spices are beginning to brown, add the chopped tomato – stand back, as the water in the juice will make the oil spit. Give it all a good stir before scraping the tarka into the dal. Cover with a lid and cook for a few minutes. Stir again, check the seasoning, then serve with the boiled rice.

Note:
- For a complete meal, this works well with Cauliflower 'Rice' and Indian Salad (see pages 177 and 144).

Braised Puy Lentils with Bay Leaves
Serves 4

> *olive oil spray*
> *1 medium onion, peeled and roughly chopped*
> *500 g (1 lb 2 oz) carrots, peeled and sliced*
> *500 g (1 lb 2 oz) leeks, trimmed and cut into thick rounds*
> *2 bay leaves*
> *2 fresh thyme sprigs*
> *250 g (9 oz) Puy lentils*
> *400 g (14 oz) can chopped tomatoes*
> *3 garlic cloves, peeled and crushed*
> *salt and freshly ground black pepper*
> *chopped fresh parsley, to garnish*

Spray a few squirts of olive oil spray in a large pan and set over the heat. Add the onion and cook gently for about 10 minutes, until translucent. Add the carrots, leeks, bay leaves and thyme and cook for a further 10 minutes. Stir in the Puy lentils and add 1 litre (1¾ pints) cold water. Bring to the boil and cook for 30–40 minutes until the lentils are cooked through. Add the canned tomatoes and garlic and cook for a further 10 minutes. Season with salt and pepper to taste. Serve topped with a sprinkle of chopped parsley.

Note:
- This would make a lovely filling for a vegan cottage pie, either topped with traditional mash or with our White Bean Mash (see page 180).

Stuffed Peppers
Serves 4

olive oil spray
4 peppers, red or yellow, halved vertically and deseeded
200 g (7 oz) basmati rice, rinsed
75 g (2½ oz) shallots, peeled and finely chopped
2 large garlic cloves, peeled and finely chopped
100 g (3½ oz) celery, trimmed and finely chopped
1 tsp fennel seeds
125 g (4 oz) chestnut mushrooms, wiped and finely
  chopped
25 g (1 oz) sultanas
35 g (1¼ oz) pine nuts, pan-roasted
1 tsp dried chilli flakes
salt and freshly ground black pepper

Preheat the oven to 180°C/350°F/Gas mark 4.

Spray or wipe the pepper halves with olive oil spray and place in a roasting tin or dish.

Cook the rice for about 20 minutes or until just done – al dente – then drain and leave to cool.

Spray a few squirts of olive oil spray in a large pan and set over a low heat. When hot, add the shallots and garlic and gently fry until soft. Add the celery and fennel seeds then mushrooms and cook for 15 minutes. When cooked through, add the sultanas, pine nuts and chilli flakes and cook for a further 5 minutes. Mix everything together with the cooled rice, then season with salt, adding a generous grinding of black pepper. Spoon the filling into the pepper halves, pressing down well and bake in the oven for 20–25 minutes. Serve with any remaining rice mixture alongside.

LIGHT MEALS, SIDE DISHES, DIPS AND STOCKS

Quick Quinoa Pilaf
Serves 1

2 spring onions, trimmed
½ tsp ground cumin
100 g (3½ oz) quinoa, rinsed
1 x 15 g (½ oz) sachet miso soup paste
40 g (1½ oz) green beans, trimmed and chopped into thirds
40 g (1½ oz) frozen peas

Chop the spring onions, then dry-fry in a saucepan for a minute or two. Add the cumin and the quinoa, stir and dry-fry for 2 more minutes until it starts to smell nutty. Dissolve the miso soup paste in 200 ml (7 fl oz) boiling water, then add to the quinoa together with the green beans and the frozen peas. Cover with a lid and simmer over a low heat for 20 minutes. Keep checking it doesn't boil dry; add small amounts of water if it does. When the beans are tender and the quinoa has become translucent and the pilaf is done.

Note:
• Add a handful of canned chickpeas or cooked greens at the end if desired.

Peppers Piedmontese
Serves 2

2 red, orange or yellow peppers
1 garlic clove, peeled
4 olives
4 fresh basil leaves
2 small tomatoes, halved
olive oil spray
salt and freshly ground black pepper

Preheat the oven to 180°C/350°F/Gas mark 4.

Cut each pepper in half lengthways, slicing through the stalk but leaving it attached to the pepper and arrange in a baking dish. Slice the garlic clove and divide these slices among the upturned peppers. Slice the olives and divide these among the peppers. Place a basil leaf in each pepper, followed by the halved tomatoes, cut side down. Spray with olive oil, season, and bake in the oven for 20–30 minutes.

Note:
- This can easily be scaled up to serve more people and makes a lovely accompaniment to a summer lunch or barbecue.

French Lettuce, Peas and Mint
Serves 2 as an accompaniment

3 spring onions, trimmed and chopped
250 ml (9 fl oz) vegetable stock (see page 186 or use a
good alternative such as Marigold bouillon powder)
1 Little Gem lettuce, shredded
300 g (11 oz) frozen peas
few fresh mint leaves, chopped
salt and freshly ground black pepper

In a large, wide pan, cook the spring onions in 1–2 tbsp of stock for 5 minutes. Add the lettuce, peas, mint and the remaining stock and bring to the boil. Cook briskly for 5 minutes, or until the vegetables are tender. Season with salt and pepper to taste and serve.

Cauliflower 'Rice'

Serves 2

1 small cauliflower, trimmed

Using the large holes of a cheese grater, grate the raw cauliflower into a bowl. Heat a non-stick frying pan over a medium heat, add the cauliflower and dry-fry for about 5 minutes, or until the 'rice' is beginning to soften and brown. Serve with curry as a substitute for white rice.

Spicy Bulgur Wheat and Pea Pilaf
Serves 2

olive oil spray
1 medium onion, peeled and finely chopped
½ tsp ground cumin
200 g (7 oz) bulgur wheat or quinoa, rinsed
350 ml (12 fl oz) vegetable stock (see page 186 or use a
  good alternative such as Marigold bouillon powder)
1 tbsp tomato purée
150 g (5 oz) frozen peas
1 tbsp lemon juice
salt and freshly ground black pepper

Spray or wipe the base of a shallow, lidded pan with olive oil and set over a medium heat. When hot, add the onion and stir-fry for 10 minutes or until browned. Add the cumin, followed by the bulgur wheat or quinoa. Pour in the stock and stir in the tomato purée. Cover with a lid, reduce the heat and cook slowly for about 10 minutes for bulgur wheat or 20 minutes for quinoa. When the grain is cooked, add the frozen peas leaving them on top of the grains in the pan. Replace the cover and steam the peas for a further 5 minutes, until cooked. Stir, sprinkle with the lemon juice and season with salt and pepper to taste.

Notes:
- This dish can be used to stuff peppers or tomatoes and is ideal to prepare as it's quick and easy.
- It's also portable, so is perfect for picnics or packed lunches.

Simple Bulgur Wheat Supper
Serves 2

100 g (3½ oz) bulgur wheat
275 ml (9 fl oz) vegetable stock (see page 186 or use a
good alternative such as Marigold bouillon powder)
3 medium tomatoes
salt and freshly ground black pepper
balsamic vinegar, for drizzling
4 tbsp canned haricot beans
fresh flat-leaf parsley and chives, finely chopped, to taste

Preheat the grill to medium.

Put the bulgur wheat and stock in a medium-sized bowl and leave for about 15 minutes until all the liquid has been absorbed.

Meanwhile, halve the tomatoes and put them in a dish that can be put under the grill. Season the tomatoes with a little salt and pepper, then put under the grill for about 5 minutes, or until soft. Top with a drizzle of balsamic vinegar and crush gently with a fork. Set aside.

Once the bulgur is ready to eat, fluff up the grains with a fork, then add the beans, and mix together with finely chopped herbs to taste. Season with salt and pepper and serve the bean and bulgur mix with the grilled tomatoes.

White Bean Mash
Serves 2 as an accompaniment

400 g (14 oz) can white beans (cannellini work well)
½ medium onion, peeled and finely chopped
1 tbsp finely chopped fresh herbs, such as rosemary or
* thyme*
salt and freshly ground black pepper

Pour the beans into a small saucepan, together with the liquid from the can. Add the onion and herbs and simmer over a medium heat for 5 minutes.

Drain the mixture and return to the saucepan. Using a potato masher, mash the beans coarsely. Season to taste and serve.

Avocado Toast
Serves 1

1 slice of bread, preferably wholegrain
1 tbsp houmous
½ perfectly ripe avocado
salt and freshly ground black pepper
a wedge of lemon

Toast the bread. Spread with the houmous, then slice or mash the avocado and place on top of the houmous. Season with salt and pepper, and a squeeze of lemon juice if required.

Broccoli with Chilli
Serves 2

1 head of broccoli
olive oil spray
2 garlic cloves, peeled and sliced
1 mild red chilli, sliced
salt and freshly ground black pepper

Break up the broccoli into individual, even-sized florets. Cook the florets in a pan of boiling water for 3 minutes only, before draining and plunging into cold water. Oil a frying pan or wok and set over the heat. Add the sliced garlic and chilli, 1 tbsp water and the drained broccoli, and stir-fry until the broccoli is browned and tender. Taste for seasoning and serve.

Note:
• Avoid burning the garlic as it will become bitter.

Roasted Cauliflower with Cumin
Serves 2

1 head of cauliflower
olive oil spray
1 tsp cumin seeds
salt and freshly ground black pepper

Preheat the oven to 220°C/425°F/Gas mark 7 and line a baking tray with baking parchment.

Break up the head of cauliflower into individual florets and spray with olive oil spray. Put the cumin seeds, seasoning and 1 tbsp water in a large bowl. Tip in the florets and stir to coat well. Pour the cauliflower mixture on to the lined baking tray, spreading out the florets and cook in the oven for 20–30 minutes, turning occasionally. When the cauliflower is nicely browned and tender, transfer to a serving dish and serve.

Note:
- This is a lovely way to add flavour to a vegetable that isn't always very tasty. On a Moderation Day, serve this with a minty yogurt dip made by mixing Greek yogurt with chopped mint and cucumber, and sprinkled with pomegranate seeds.

Pumpkin Seeds with Soy Sauce
Serves 1

handful of pumpkin or sunflower seeds, or a mixture of both
enough soy sauce (or Tamari or Japanese teriyaki sauce) to coat the seeds

Preheat the oven to 180°C/350°F/Gas mark 4.

Coat the seeds well in the soy sauce. You could also add chilli flakes or cumin seeds at this stage. Lay the seeds out on a non-stick baking tray and roast in the oven for about 10 minutes. Keep an eye on the seeds while they are in the oven as they may burn. Leave to cool and serve.

Note:
• Seeds are nutrient dense, making this recipe a good one for salad toppings or a snack on the go.

Butternut Squash and Rosewater Dip
Makes about 750 ml–1 litre (1¼–1¾ pints)

> 1 medium butternut squash, peeled and deseeded and
>   cut into chunks
> 3 garlic cloves, peeled and crushed
> 2 tbsp lemon juice
> 1 tbsp tahini (sesame seed paste)
> 1 tsp rosewater
> 1 tsp honey
> salt and freshly ground black pepper

Preheat the oven to 200°C/400°F/Gas mark 6 and line a baking tray with baking parchment.

Place the squash chunks on the lined baking tray and bake in the oven for 20 minutes, or until soft. Remove from the oven, place in a blender or food processor with the remaining ingredients and whizz to a smooth consistency, adding a little warm water to loosen the dip if it's too thick. Season with salt and pepper to taste.

Note:
- Serve with crudités for a delicious starter or a healthy party snack, or use as a sandwich filling or toast topping for a quick Fast Day lunch with crisp salad to top.

Vegetable Stock
Makes 1.5 litres (2½ pints)

4 large carrots, peeled and cut into large pieces

2 medium leeks, carefully washed, trimmed and roughly chopped

2 large (or 3 medium) onions, peeled and roughly chopped

2 celery sticks, trimmed and roughly chopped

2 garlic cloves, crushed, peeled and chopped

½ lemon, halved again

1 star anise

1 bouquet garni, or herbs of your choice (go easy on the thyme)

1 bay leaf

6 black peppercorns

Put all the ingredients into a large saucepan or stockpot. Cover with 2 litres (3½ pints) water and bring to a simmer, leaving to bubble away gently for 1½–2 hours. Top up with water as needed, keeping the ingredients covered at all times.

Notes:
- Do not add salt to the stock; that comes later, when you are using it to make soups, casseroles or tagines. Strain, cool, and refrigerate or freeze if you are not using immediately.
- This stock can be made in bulk and refrigerated for several days. It will form the base of all your vegetable soups. The first four ingredients are integral to a good stock; the others you can vary according to taste and availability.

CHAPTER 18

MODERATION DAY RECIPES

BREAKFASTS

Bircher Muesli Breakfast Pot
Serves 1

¼ *medium banana*
5 strawberries
2 tbsp apple juice
250 g (9 oz) Greek yogurt
3 tbsp porridge (rolled) oats

Mash together the banana, strawberries and apple juice. Stir into the Greek yogurt together with the oats. Store in the fridge for up to 24 hours before eating.

Note:
- Make this the night before and store in a jam jar in the fridge, for a quick or on-the-go breakfast the following day.

Huevos Rancheros
Serves 2

2 large free-range eggs
1 tsp semi-skimmed milk
½ small red chilli, finely sliced or chopped, to taste
salt and freshly ground black pepper
chopped fresh coriander, to garnish

To serve:
slices of ripe avocado
1–2 tbsp tomato salsa
a small amount of low-fat refried beans or leftover
  Black Bean Chilli (see page 163)

Break the eggs into a bowl, add the milk and whisk together to combine. Add the chilli and salt and pepper to taste.

Heat a non-stick pan and add the eggs, using a spatula to keep moving the mixture around. Once scrambled, remove the pan from the heat and serve with your choice of avocado slices, tomato salsa, refried beans or leftover Black Bean Chilli, and garnish with fresh coriander.

Note:
• For a substantial breakfast or a light lunch, serve this with a toasted corn tortilla.

Scrambled Egg with Rye Toast
Serves 2

> *5 large free-range eggs*
> *ground white pepper*
> *1 large, or 2 small, slices of rye bread, cut reasonably*
> *thick*
> *1 tbsp unsalted butter*
> *salt, if required*

Break 4 whole eggs and 1 egg yolk, into a small mixing bowl and mix thoroughly, until they become a uniform yellow colour. Add a small amount of white pepper and mix well. Do not add salt.

Toast the rye bread. Heat the butter gently in a small, non-stick saucepan; do not allow to burn. Once melted, add the eggs and start to stir gently. As the egg mixture starts to cook on the base of the pan, scrape it off, mixing it back into the uncooked egg. Continue to do this, stopping just before the eggs are cooked through (they are still a little runny and look slightly underdone). Remove the pan from the heat and set aside. The eggs will have gently continued to cook in the pan, so add salt if required, stir in and serve immediately.

Banana and Blueberry Smoothie
Serves 1

100 g (3 oz) Greek yogurt
150 ml (5 fl oz) milk (semi-skimmed or skimmed)
1 ripe banana
large handful of blueberries
½ tsp vanilla extract (optional)

Whizz all the ingredients to your desired consistency in a blender, adding more milk if required.

Greek Yogurt with Granola and Fruit
Serves 1

250 g (9 oz) Greek yogurt
handful of sugar-free muesli or granola or rolled oats
fresh fruit, such as berries
honey, if desired

Put the yogurt into a bowl and layer with the muesli or granola, fruit and a tiny amount of honey. Eat right away.

Note:
- If you are not used to eating natural yogurt it can seem very plain. A dash of vanilla essence or a sprinkle of ground cinnamon/mixed spice livens it up.

Banana Pancakes
Serves 1

1 medium banana
1 large free-range egg, beaten
pinch of ground cinnamon
vegetable oil spray

Mash the banana and mix with the beaten egg, then add the cinnamon. Heat a heavy-based saucepan, drizzle with a flavourless oil, then pour in the banana/egg mixture and cook until golden brown and firm on one side, about 3 minutes. Flip over and cook for about 2 minutes or until browned. Serve immediately.

Note:
• This is delicious served with fresh berries.

Poached Eggs

salt

eggs, preferably organic and as fresh as possible, 1 per person

vinegar, any type will do but clear white vinegar is preferable

slices of thick rye bread, toasted, to serve

Bring a medium-sized pan of well-salted water to simmering point. Crack 1 egg into a teacup or small jug and add ½ tsp vinegar. Create a whirlpool in the pan of simmering water by stirring vigorously with a balloon whisk. The water will form a deep vortex; lower the cup into the water, just below the surface and quickly tip the egg in. The egg should swirl around, forming an oval shape. Reduce the heat and cook for 3 minutes. When done, serve immediately on a thick slice of rye bread toast.

Note:

- Poaching is a simple way of cooking eggs so that they retain all their natural flavour. If cooking several eggs, do them one at a time and when each is cooked drop it gently into a bowl of iced water, with added ice cubes. This will suspend the cooking process. When ready to serve, reheat the chilled eggs in a pan of simmering water for 30 seconds.

SALADS

Hearty Harissa Salad

(See page 140, Fast Day) with Greek Yogurt Dressing

Greek Salad

Serves 4

2 large tomatoes
1 medium cucumber, peeled
120 g (4 oz) feta cheese
1 red onion, peeled and thinly sliced into fine rings
10 Kalamata olives
1 tbsp olive oil
½ tbsp red wine vinegar
pinch of dried oregano
salt and freshly ground black pepper

Slice each tomato into 8 wedges. Slice the cucumber length-ways before chopping each half into thin slices. Use a fork to break up the cheese into bite-sized chunks. In a bowl, combine the tomatoes, cucumber, onion, olives and cheese. In a small cup, combine the oil, vinegar, oregano and salt and pepper. Whisk the dressing before pouring over the salad. Serve immediately.

Note:

• A classic Greek salad, this has a little less of the usual quantity of dressing. Serve with crusty bread.

Mackerel Salad

Serves 4

> *2 x 125 g (4 oz) cans mackerel in tomato sauce*
>   *(or sardines)*
> *400 g (14 oz) can cannellini beans*
> *crisp salad leaves*
> *250 g (9 oz) cherry tomatoes*

Warm the mackerel and beans slightly in a pan, if desired, breaking up the fish while you do so. Serve with the salad leaves and tomatoes on the side or toss all the ingredients together if using the mackerel and beans at room temperature.

SOUPS

Chicken Soup
Serves 4

1 large carrot, peeled and diced
2 celery sticks, trimmed and diced
1 small onion, peeled, halved and sliced
1 small sweet potato, peeled and diced
1 tsp olive oil
500 ml (18 fl oz) fresh chicken stock
1 bouquet garni
1 bay leaf
125 g (4 oz) chopped cooked chicken breast

Sauté the vegetables in the olive oil for about 15 minutes, or until translucent. Add the stock and herbs and simmer until all the vegetables are cooked. Add the chicken and simmer until piping hot. Remove the herbs before serving.

Note:
• This is a great way to use up leftover roast chicken.

Sri Lankan Sweet Potato Soup
Serves 4

1 tsp olive oil

1 red onion, peeled and chopped

2 garlic cloves, peeled and finely sliced

1 tsp each of cumin seeds, coriander seeds and sesame seeds

2-cm (¾-in) piece of fresh ginger, peeled and thinly sliced

1 green chilli, deseeded and thinly sliced

1.5 litres (2½ pints) vegetable stock (see page 186 or use a good alternative such as Marigold bouillon powder)

1 lime, quartered

350 g (12 oz) sweet potato, peeled and cubed

350 g (12 oz) butternut squash, or other variety of squash, peeled, deseeded and cut into 1-cm (½-in) cubes

1 tbsp roughly chopped fresh coriander leaves, plus extra whole leaves to garnish

salt and freshly ground black pepper

Greek yogurt, to serve

Heat the oil in a large pan, add the onion and cook gently for 10 minutes, or until translucent. Add the garlic, spices, ginger and chilli, then stir well and cook for a further 5 minutes.

Add the stock, lime, sweet potato, squash and coriander leaves. Bring to a simmer and cook for about 15–20 minutes. Taste for seasoning and add salt and pepper as needed. Serve with a swirl of Greek yogurt and top with a sprinkle of coriander leaves.

Coriander and Coconut Soup
Serves 4

> 600 ml (1 pint) fresh chicken or vegetable stock (see
>   page 186 or use a good alternative such as Marigold
>   bouillon powder)
> 1–2 Tom Yam stock cubes or green Thai curry paste, to taste
> 2-cm (¾-in) piece fresh galangal root, peeled and
>   roughly chopped
> 6 spring onions or shallots, trimmed or peeled and finely
>   chopped
> 2 lemongrass stalks, white part only, crushed
> 1 garlic clove, peeled and crushed
> large bunch of fresh coriander, leaves reserved, stalks
>   chopped
> 400 g (14 oz) can coconut milk
> juice of 1 lime
> 2 kaffir lime leaves
> few Thai basil leaves (optional)
> 1 tbsp Thai fish sauce (nam pla), or more to taste
> thin strips of chicken, fish or large prawns (optional)
> whole red bird's-eye chillies, to garnish

Simmer the stock, stock cube or curry paste, galangal, onions, lemongrass and garlic in a large pan for 30 minutes. Sieve, put into a blender or food processor with the coriander stalks and blend thoroughly. Strain into the rinsed-out pan, add the coconut milk, lime juice, lime leaves, Thai basil leaves and fish sauce and reheat for 5 minutes. Add the chicken, fish or prawns, heat for a further 10–15 minutes. Garnish with bird's-eye chillies, sprinkle with the remaining coriander leaves and serve.

MAIN MEALS: STEWS, PASTA AND BAKES

Mount Athos Baked Fish
Serves 6

4 large onions, peeled and sliced
6 white fish fillets, such as cod or haddock
8 garlic cloves, peeled but left whole
150 ml (5 fl oz) olive oil
salt and freshly ground black pepper
2 tbsp finely chopped fresh parsley

Preheat the oven to 180°C/350°F/Gas mark 4.

Put the onion slices in a large pan and cover with water. Bring to the boil then reduce the heat and simmer for 30 minutes. Drain the onions, making sure you retain the liquid and discard the onions. Arrange the fish and garlic in a large ovenproof dish, and pour the onion liquid and the olive oil over the top. Season with salt and pepper and bake in the oven for 25 minutes, or until the fish is cooked. Serve sprinkled with the chopped parsley and with the cooking juices poured over.

Tunisian Fish Tagine
Serves 4

1 tbsp olive oil
2 shallots, peeled and chopped
500 ml (18 fl oz) fish or chicken stock, or water
½ tsp saffron threads
2 garlic cloves, peeled and crushed
½ green chilli, finely sliced, plus extra to serve
2-cm (¾-in) piece of fresh ginger, peeled and grated
1 tbsp tomato purée
2 tsp ground cumin
1 tsp ground coriander
1 tsp ground cinnamon
2 tbsp ground almonds
8–10 cherry tomatoes, halved
1 small lemon, quartered or better still, a preserved
  lemon, thickly sliced
1 tbsp honey
750 g (1 lb 10 oz) firm white fish, such as monkfish,
  haddock, halibut or bass, cut into large chunks
small bunch of fresh coriander, roughly chopped,
  including the stalks
handful of toasted flaked almonds

Heat the olive oil in the tagine base, add the shallots and cook slowly for 10 minutes until translucent.

Meanwhile, heat the stock or water in another pan and add the saffron. When the shallots are cooked through, add the garlic, chilli and ginger and cook for a further 5 minutes. Add the tomato purée and all the spices and cook for a further

2 minutes. Add the ground almonds, tomatoes, lemon quarters, honey and saffron-soaked stock, put the tagine lid on and simmer gently for 10 minutes to thicken the sauce, by which time the tomatoes will have started to break up. Cook a little longer if the sauce is too thin. At this stage you can stop the cooking process, or keep in the fridge overnight if you wish, adding the remaining ingredients later.

Reheat the sauce, if necessary, and add the fish. Mix well into the sauce, making sure all the fish is well covered. Simmer for 5 minutes then check the fish to make sure it is cooked. For an extra fresh burst of flavour, scatter over some more sliced chilli. Finally, sprinkle over the coriander and toasted almonds and serve.

Note:
• Serve with couscous or brown rice, and natural yogurt.

Chicken Tagine
Serves 4

1 tbsp olive oil
4 skinless, boneless chicken thighs
1 large onion, peeled and thinly sliced
3 cloves garlic, peeled and thinly sliced
3 tsp grated fresh ginger
2 tsp paprika
1 tsp turmeric
2 tsp ground cumin
1 tsp cayenne pepper
1 tsp ground cinnamon
300 g (11 oz) can chickpeas, drained
400 g (14 oz) can chopped tomatoes
1 tbsp honey
salt and freshly ground black pepper
1 tbsp pine nuts
handful of chopped fresh coriander leaves, to garnish

Heat the olive oil in tagine base and brown the chicken pieces, then remove from the tagine and set aside.

In the same oil, add the onion and cook gently until soft and translucent. Add the garlic, ginger and all the spices and cook through for 3 minutes. Stir in 100 ml (3½ fl oz) water or chicken stock, then add the reserved chicken pieces, chickpeas, tomatoes and honey and season with salt and pepper. Replace the lid and simmer gently for 10–15 minutes, adding more water or stock if needed.

Meanwhile, carefully toast the pine nuts in a dry frying pan until golden. Adjust the tagine seasoning if necessary. Garnish with pine nuts and chopped coriander, and serve.

Asian Poached Chicken with Sesame Green Beans
Serves 4

1 medium onion, peeled and roughly chopped

3 star anise

1 cinnamon stick

2-cm (¾-in) piece of fresh ginger, peeled and thinly sliced

2 lemongrass stalks, well crushed

2 small red chillies, deseeded and thinly sliced

2 tbsp light soy sauce

1 tbsp Thai fish sauce (nam pla)

small bunch of fresh coriander, roughly chopped

500 ml (18 fl oz) chicken stock or vegetable stock (see page 186 or use a good alternative such as Marigold bouillon powder)

4 skinless chicken breast fillets, thickly sliced

500 g (1 lb 2 oz) green beans, cut into 5-cm (2-in) pieces

1 tbsp sesame seeds

1 garlic clove, peeled and very finely chopped

chopped fresh coriander leaves, to garnish

Combine the first 10 ingredients in a large saucepan and bring to a gentle simmer. Add the chicken slices and cook for 15 minutes, then remove the pan from the heat and leave the chicken in the liquid to cool.

Strain some of the chicken cooking juices into a separate pan, add the beans and boil for about 5 minutes, until just tender (there should be a little residual 'bite' to keep them crunchy).

Heat a frying pan and dry-fry the sesame seeds and chopped garlic until golden, keeping an eye on them to stop them burning, then combine the drained beans with the sesame seeds and garlic.

Serve the chicken together with the sauce and the beans, and garnish with chopped coriander leaves.

Note:

• This is best served with a small jacket potato, as the potato really soaks up the sauce.

Spaghetti with Leeks and Butternut Squash
Serves 4

1 large butternut squash, peeled and roughly chopped
200 g (7 oz) wholewheat spaghetti
olive oil spray
1 medium leek, white part only, finely chopped
2 garlic cloves, peeled and crushed
5 fresh sage leaves, finely chopped
30 g (1¼ oz) Parmesan cheese, grated, plus extra to
  serve (optional)
salt and freshly ground black pepper

Boil a large pan of water and add the butternut squash chunks. Cook until soft, about 10 minutes, then remove from the pan with a slotted spoon (reserving the pan and water for cooking the spaghetti) and place in a bowl. Add the pasta to the pan and cook according to the packet instructions. Blend the squash using a hand-held stick blender or potato masher, until it is a purée.

Spray a little olive oil spray in a large pan and set over a medium heat. Add the leeks and crushed garlic and sauté until soft and beginning to brown. Add the squash purée together with the sage and Parmesan, then season with salt and pepper. If the sauce is too thick, use a little of the pasta water to thin it down. Once cooked add the drained spaghetti to the sauce and stir well. Serve with a little more Parmesan, if desired.

Note:
• This works well with other types of squash, too, so it's worth experimenting with different vegetable purées as sauces.

Thai-style Bean Patties with Spicy Pepper Dipping Sauce

Serves 2 as a main course or 4 as a side dish

400 g (14 oz) can cannellini beans
2 spring onions, trimmed and finely chopped
2 kaffir lime leaves, finely chopped with stems removed
handful of chopped fresh coriander leaves
2–3 tsp red or green Thai curry paste
salt and freshly ground black pepper
250 g (9 oz) plain flour
1 large free-range egg, whisked
50 g (1¾ oz) breadcrumbs or ground almonds
2 tbsp olive oil
lime wedges, to serve

Spicy Pepper Dipping Sauce:
2 red, orange or yellow peppers (not green), deseeded
  and chopped
3 tsp pomegranate molasses
1½ tsp rice vinegar or white wine vinegar
1 tsp chilli flakes or 2 small bird's-eye chillies, finely
  chopped

Drain the cannellini beans, rinse and dry well in a clean tea towel. Put the beans into a bowl and add the spring onions, lime leaves, coriander, Thai curry paste and salt to taste. Mix thoroughly, transfer to a food processor and whizz until a firm purée forms.

For the sauce, put the peppers into a clean food processor, add the pomegranate molasses, vinegar, chilli flakes or chopped chillies and whizz until roughly chopped, adding a little water if needed. Set aside.

Spread the flour out on a plate, put the beaten egg into a shallow bowl and spread the breadcrumbs or ground almonds out in another bowl. Using your hands, form the bean mixture into 2–4 patties, then coat in the flour, dip into the beaten egg and roll carefully in the breadcrumbs or almonds.

Heat the olive oil in a small frying pan over a medium heat and fry the bean cakes for about 5 minutes on each side until golden, turning once. Serve with lemon wedges and the dipping sauce on the side.

Note:
• This is also lovely served with rocket salad and dressing and lime wedges.

Monastery Vegetable Bake
Serves 4

1 tbsp dried oregano
1 tbsp finely chopped fresh mint
2 garlic cloves, crushed and chopped
400 g (14 oz) can chopped tomatoes
1 medium onion, peeled and roughly chopped
2 medium aubergines, trimmed and cut into 2.5-cm
    (1-in) cubes
2 tbsp olive oil
500 g (1 lb 2 oz) potatoes, thinly sliced
200 g (7 oz) feta cheese, cubed
salt and freshly ground black pepper

Preheat the oven to 200°C/400°F/Gas mark 6.

Mix the oregano, mint, garlic and tomatoes together in a pan and simmer gently for about 15 minutes.

In a separate pan, cook the onion and aubergines gently in the olive oil for about 10 minutes until the onions are translucent. When cooked, arrange the vegetables in an ovenproof dish, layer the sliced potatoes on top, then the feta cheese, and finally spread over the tomato sauce, seasoning each layer as you go.

Bake in the oven for about 45 minutes. Check after 30 minutes and if the top layer looks as if it is drying out, or threatening to burn, cover the dish with foil. Leave to cool for 10–15 minutes before eating.

Note:
• Serve with a green salad.

Poached Salmon with Fennel
Serves 4

4 salmon fillets, skin removed
1 fennel bulb, trimmed and thinly sliced
1 medium red onion, peeled and very thinly sliced
250–350 ml (9–12 fl oz) dry white wine, such as Pinot
  Grigio or Sauvignon Blanc
juice and zest of 1 medium orange
1 tbsp capers, rinsed and drained
salt and ground white pepper

Preheat the oven to 180°C/350°F/Gas mark 4.

Using foil, make 4 parcels by cutting the foil into squares, each large enough to hold the salmon fillets, fennel, onion and wine. Place 1 fillet and a quarter each of the sliced fennel and onion in the centre of each foil square. Lift up the 4 sides of the foil to form parcels. Before closing the top, pour over white wine, then add 1 tbsp orange juice, some orange zest and a sprinkling of capers and finish by adding salt and just a pinch of white pepper. Close the top of the parcel, folding over to make a tight seal, then place on a baking tray and bake on the middle shelf of the oven. After 30 minutes, check one of the parcels to see if the salmon is done. It should be springy to the touch. Remove from the oven and transfer the salmon and vegetables to a separate serving dish. Pour the cooking juices into a small saucepan and boil vigorously to reduce to a syrupy consistency. If there are insufficient juices left after baking, top up with extra wine. Pour over the sauce and serve.

Note:
• This is a substantial main meal when served with green beans and boiled new potatoes.

Pasta with Rocket
Serves 2

170 g (6 oz) pasta, such as tagliatelle, fettucine,
* pappardelle or other thin ribbon pasta*
1 tbsp olive oil
½ fresh or dried red chilli, chopped
1 garlic clove, peeled and chopped
generous handful of rocket
salt and freshly ground black pepper
Parmesan cheese, to serve (optional)

Bring a large pan of water to the boil. Add the pasta and cook according the packet instructions until it is al dente.

Meanwhile, heat the olive oil in a separate pan and gently sauté the chilli and garlic for 2 minutes. Add the rocket and stir through. Test the pasta and when al dente, remove from the pan and drain well. Put the pasta back into the pan, add the rocket mixture, stir through and season well. Serve in bowls topped with a tiny shaving of Parmesan, if desired.

LIGHTER MEALS AND SIMPLE SUPPERS

Grilled Lemon Salmon

Serves 4

olive oil, for brushing
4 salmon fillets
1 lemon, halved
1 tbsp capers, drained and rinsed
finely chopped parsley, for sprinkling
finely chopped chives, for sprinkling
salt and freshly ground black pepper

Preheat the grill to medium.

Using a pastry brush, brush a small amount of oil over each side of the salmon fillets. Place under the grill, along with the lemon halves, cut side down, and grill for about 5 minutes on each side, or until firm. Transfer the fish to a serving plate and squeeze over a little of the lemon juice. Sprinkle with the capers and herbs, and season with salt and pepper.

Moroccan Roast Chicken Salad
Serves 6

1 kg (2¼ lb) chicken breast, skinned and sliced
salt and freshly ground black pepper
2 tbsp olive oil
1 large orange
50 g (1¾ oz) runny honey
½ tsp saffron threads
1 tbsp white wine vinegar
2 tbsp virgin olive oil
1 large or 2 small fennel bulbs, trimmed and finely
  sliced
25 g (1 oz) fresh coriander leaves, lightly chopped
25 g (1 oz) fresh basil leaves, torn
25 g (1 oz) fresh flat-leaf parsley, roughly chopped
2 tbsp lemon juice
1 red chilli, finely sliced
1 garlic clove, peeled and crushed

Preheat the oven to 200°C/400°F/Gas mark 6.

Season the chicken breasts well. Heat a frying pan until very hot, add half of the olive oil and sear the chicken for 1–2 minutes on each side, until browned. Transfer to a roasting tin and roast in the oven for 15–20 minutes, or until just cooked. Do not overcook. Remove from the oven and leave to cool. Tear the chicken into large chunks and set aside.

Meanwhile, cut off the top and bottom of the orange and cut, skin on, into 10–12 wedges (the more the better). Remove any pips and place in a non-stick saucepan with the honey, saffron threads and vinegar. Add enough water, about 300–400 ml

(10–14 fl oz), to cover the orange wedges. Bring to the boil, then reduce the heat to low and very gently simmer for up to 1 hour, or when the sauce reaches the consistency of a thick syrup. Add a little more water during cooking if the liquid level gets too low. You are aiming for around 5 tbsp syrup.

Place the orange wedges with their syrup into a food processor or blender and whizz to a thin paste, adding more water if needed.

Place the shredded chicken in a large mixing bowl, add half the orange paste and stir well. Add the remaining ingredients to the chicken and stir until well mixed. Drizzle with the remaining olive oil. Add more oil or lemon juice if needed.

Note:
- Any remaining orange paste can be refrigerated or frozen for future use.

Baked Sweet Potatoes with Olives and Feta
Serves 2

2 medium sweet potatoes
100 g (3½ oz) feta cheese
10 Kalamata olives
salt and freshly ground black pepper
chilli flakes, to taste
green salad, to serve

Preheat the oven to 200°C/400°F/Gas mark 6.

Place the sweet potatoes on a rack in the oven, with a baking tray underneath to catch any drips and bake for 30 minutes, or until they are soft all the way through.

Meanwhile, break up the feta cheese with a fork, halve the olives, taking out any stones, and mix together in a bowl with seasoning and chilli flakes, to taste. When the potatoes are cooked, halve lengthways and fill with the feta and olives. Serve with a large green salad.

Egg Fried Rice
Serves 2

1 tsp sunflower oil
½ onion, peeled and finely chopped
3 spring onions, trimmed and chopped
1 garlic clove, peeled and crushed
1-cm (½-in) piece of fresh ginger, peeled and finely chopped
1 carrot, peeled and cut into matchsticks
1 red or yellow pepper, cored and finely sliced
50 g (1¾ oz) frozen peas
50 g (1¾ oz) frozen sweetcorn
75 g (2½ oz) broccoli, cut into small pieces
2 cups cold cooked rice
1 egg
soy sauce, to taste

Heat the oil in a large frying pan or wok. When hot, add the onion, spring onions, garlic and ginger and stir-fry briskly for 2 minutes. Add the carrot, pepper, peas, sweetcorn and broccoli and stir-fry until browned and soft. Add the cold cooked rice and begin to combine with the vegetables. Move this mixture to one side in the pan while you crack in the egg and quickly scramble it. When cooked and beginning to brown, mix in the rice and vegetable mixture. Add soy sauce to taste and serve.

Note:
- This is a great way to use up vegetables and you can substitute most vegetables in this dish. Kids really enjoy this one, too.

DESSERTS

Baked Apples
Serves 1

For each person:
1 tbsp raisins
a grating of fresh lemon zest
1 tsp maple syrup
¼ tsp ground cinnamon
1 large eating apple

Preheat the oven to 175°C/347°F/Gas mark 3.

Mix together the first four ingredients. Core the apple and score a line round the middle of the apple with a knife (this prevents the apple from splitting during baking). Place the apple on a baking tray and insert the raisin mixture into the core area. Bake in the oven for 30–40 minutes, or until cooked.

Note:
• Serve with a small amount of Greek yogurt for Moderation Days.

Pineapple, Berry and Mint Fruit Salad
Serves 4

1 pineapple, peeled and chopped into bite-size pieces
1 mango, peeled, stoned and chopped into bite-size
*   pieces*
200 g (7 oz) blueberries
200 g (7 oz) raspberries
fresh mint leaves
honey, to taste

Place all the fruit into a bowl and mix together. Tear over mint leaves and drizzle a small amount of honey on top.

Melon with Rosewater
Serves 2

1 ripe honeydew or cantaloupe melon
1 tsp rosewater

Slice the melon, remove the seeds and arrange the slices on a plate. Sprinkle with the rosewater and serve.

Orange with Mint and Orange Blossom Water
Serves 2

2 large oranges
fresh mint leaves
1 tsp orange blossom water
honey, to taste (optional)

Cut off the top and bottom of the oranges. Using a sharp knife, slice away the skin before paring each orange segment away from its membrane and pith. Arrange the orange slices on a plate and sprinkle with fresh mint leaves. Drizzle over the orange blossom water and honey to taste, if desired.

Banana 'Ice Cream'
Serves 1

1 banana

Line a baking tray with baking parchment. Slice a banana and spread the slices out on the lined tray. Freeze. When frozen, put the banana slices into a food processor and whizz. At first this will sound loud but soon the slices will break down into a creamy 'ice cream'. Serve immediately.

CHAPTER 19

FEAST DAYS

One of the main reasons traditional dieting does not work is that it doesn't allow for regular indulgence. Many dieters recognise the 'binge and purge' or 'yo-yo dieting' cycle, veering from abstemious extreme to off-the-wagon disregard. The Mount Athos Diet is different as there is a regular day a week devoted to eating the sorts of foods you ate before dieting, and because it's limited to one day a week, you are unlikely to scupper your long-term progress.

Spent all week craving a piece of cake? Eat it on a Feast Day. Special occasion planned? Arrange your Mount Athos Diet week around red-letter days and festive occasions. There is absolutely no reason why you can't indulge.

All we suggest is that you think about the choices you make on a Feast Day. The temptation is to go overboard once a week, every week, and indulge in full English breakfasts, fish and chips, meals out with friends and plenty of alcohol. While the diet does not prohibit this, try to be mindful of your goals and eat accordingly.

There are different ways to approach the Feast Day, and different dieters will find their own paths. For some, it's about making a favourite meal for the family: a roast dinner, for example. For others, it's freedom to choose whatever the mood desires on that particular day.

The Mount Athos Diet authors each approach Feast Days from a different perspective:

On Saturdays, I'm out with the family. Whether we spend the day at the park, complete with picnic and perhaps an ice-cream treat, or off to see the latest kids' cinema release, I know that I can join in with the rest of the family without worrying about my diet. Children really pick up on differences and also are acutely aware of emotions. This way, I can avoid having to explain why everyone else is eating ice cream but not me, and I'd like them to see that treats can be enjoyed as just that: treats, rather than an everyday entitlement.

Often, we spend the weekend evenings with friends, and this (more often than not) revolves around a long meal with lots to drink. Since I've been on the Mount Athos Diet, my physical capacity for vast quantities of food has reduced and I rarely accept seconds, or plough through half a box of chocolates. But I'm glad to have the option there should the mood take me. This alone makes me less inclined to be greedy – knowing I could if I wanted to often means I don't.

Lottie Storey

As we have reiterated throughout this book following the principles of the Mount Athos Diet seems to result in changes in what we want to cook and eat. Before I started on the diet, meat was always a great attraction for me. I loved beef and lamb, as well as game, offal and processed meats. All this has changed. I have now been following the diet for seven months and during that time have bought and cooked beef twice and lamb once.

Our Moderation Day meals of fish and chicken have become so natural that the thought of strong meats has become off-putting. Feast Day meals are not much more indulgent than Moderation Days. We may eat more food – a starter, perhaps, or a pudding, some cheese – but they will almost always revolve around a main course of fish or chicken.

And by saving on the cost of wine throughout the week, there is the opportunity to splash out on a decent bottle of wine on our Feast Day.

Richard Storey

Friday or Saturday are usually my Feast Days, depending on what social events we have arranged. It's the day when we go out for a meal, cook for friends or go to a party. If it's a quiet weekend, then it's the day that I'll do some baking or cook a nice meal. When you like food and cooking, it's nice to have the chance to still cook with whatever ingredients you fancy every now and again.

I've noticed that I'm even more conscious of what I'm eating when I'm out than I was before. Even on a Feast Day I'm more picky about the savoury snacks that get offered round rather than just nibbling away. When you get offered food at a social event, the natural reaction is just to accept, it almost feels rude to decline. Now I think – do I really want this? Am I hungry? Often they are just cheap fried or fatty foods, so best avoided, and it's a shame to consume so many calories for something that really doesn't taste that good.

Sue Todd

Whatever your own personal approach, please allay any thoughts of guilt. The Feast Day is there to redress the balance;

to incorporate elements that on other diets spell failure. We believe this healthy equilibrium results in a more civilised approach to dieting. Emotional eating has no place on the Mount Athos Diet.

After six days of Fast and Moderation Day eating, you might well find that your taste buds have adapted and that your once favourite foods now taste too sweet or fatty. Similarly, your stomach is likely to have shrunk making the portion sizes you once ate without thought now seem colossal. These are all good signs that you are changing your eating habits for the better, for good.

At the very heart of the Mount Athos Diet is a back-to-basics approach: this is a diet focused on plenty of plant foods, meals cooked from scratch and a rejection of the high doses of salt and sugar so commonplace today. By aligning most of your week's eating to these guidelines, you are sensibly calibrating your food intake, budgeting wisely to allow for occasional splurges, and naturally adopting that 80/20 approach so often advocated as a healthy balance.

CHAPTER 20

MENU PLANNER

With the ingredients in Chapters 10 and 11, and recipes in Chapters 17 and 18, you should have everything you need to start the Mount Athos Diet. To give you a helping hand, we have devised a series of weekly menus and other suggestions, which give an idea of how the Mount Athos Diet works in practice. These menus are based on a routine of Monday, Wednesday and Friday – Fast Days, and Tuesday, Thursday and Sunday – Moderation Days. Saturdays, we are leaving you to your own devices.

WEEK 1 SAMPLE MENU

Although the Mount Athos Diet is based on the eating habits of the monks of Mount Athos, Greece, we have included a variety of recipes from around the world that adhere to the basic principles of the diet. We thought it would be good to start the Mount Athos Diet with an example menu based entirely on the Greek-style dishes in the book for your first week, complete with suggestions for accompaniments (all references to bread are without butter).

Sunday (Moderation Day)
Breakfast
Greek yogurt, granola, fruit and honey
To drink:
- Tea or coffee, small amount of milk
- Small glass of fruit juice

Lunch
Greek Salad (page 194)
Serve with:
- Small piece of bread
To drink:
- Water or small glass of fruit juice

Supper
Monastery Vegetable Bake (page 208)
Serve with:
- Salad or green vegetable
To drink:
- Up to 2 small glasses of red wine
- Water

To follow
Melon with Rosewater (page 218)
1 square of dark chocolate or other small treat

Snacks
Unlimited vegetable sticks
Limited fruit, nuts and seeds
Limited crackers or breadsticks

Monday (Fast Day)
Breakfast
Stewed Apple with Oats and syrup (page 133)
To drink:
- Black tea or coffee/herbal tea
- Water

Lunch
Mount Athos White Bean Salad (page 143)
Serve with:
- Fresh tomatoes
- Toasted pitta bread
To drink:
- Herbal tea
- Water or a small glass of fruit juice

Supper
Mount Athos Bean Soup (page 155)
Serve with:
- Small amount of wholemeal bread (no butter)
To drink:
- Herbal tea
- Water or a small glass of fruit juice

Snacks
Unlimited vegetable sticks
Limited fruit, nuts and seeds

Tuesday (Moderation Day)
Breakfast
Bircher Muesli Breakfast Pot (page 187)
Serve with:
- Fresh fruit

To drink:
- Tea or coffee, small amount of milk
- Small glass of fruit juice

Lunch
Chiucken Soup (page 196)
Serve with:
- Toasted pitta bread

To drink:
- Herbal tea
- Water or a small glass of fruit juice

Supper
Baked Sweet Potatoes with Olives and Feta (page 214)
Serve with:
- Large green salad and fresh tomatoes

To drink:
- Up to 2 small glasses of red wine
- Water

To follow
Orange with Mint and Orange Blossom Water (page 219)
1 square of dark chocolate or other small treat

Snacks
Unlimited vegetable sticks
Limited fruit, nuts and seeds
Limited crackers or breadsticks

Wednesday (Fast Day)

Breakfast
Grilled Grapefruit (page 138)
To drink:
- Black tea or coffee/herbal tea
- Water

Lunch
Mount Athos Vegetable Soup (page 153)
Serve with:
- Small amount of wholemeal bread (no butter)
To drink:
- Herbal tea
- Water or a small glass of fruit juice

Supper
Greek Baked Butter Beans (page 167)
Serve with:
- Large green salad and fresh tomatoes
To drink:
- Herbal tea
- Water or a small glass of fruit juice

Snacks
Unlimited vegetable sticks
Limited fruit, nuts and seeds

Thursday (Moderation Day)
Breakfast
Grilled Peaches with Greek yogurt (page 134)
To drink:
- Tea or coffee, small amount of milk
- Small glass of fruit juice

Lunch
Coriander and Coconut Soup (page 198)
Serve with:
- Toasted pitta bread
To drink:
- Herbal tea
- Water or a small glass of fruit juice

Supper
Hearty Harissa Salad with Greek Yogurt Dressing (page 140)
To drink:
- Up to 2 small glasses of red wine
- Water

To follow
Banana 'Ice Cream' (page 220)
1 square of dark chocolate or other small treat

Snacks
Unlimited vegetable sticks
Limited fruit, nuts and seeds
Limited crackers or breadsticks

Friday (Fast Day)

Breakfast

Muesli with Fruit Juice (page 139)

To drink:

- Black tea or coffee/herbal tea
- Water

Lunch

Mount Athos Lentil Soup (page 154)

Serve with:

- Wholemeal roll or small slice of bread

To drink:

- Herbal tea
- Water or a small glass of fruit juice

Supper

Mediterranean Ragout (page 158)

Serve with:

- Jacket potato, carrots and greens, such as cabbage, chard or kale

To drink:

- Herbal tea
- Water or a small glass of fruit juice

Snacks

Unlimited vegetable sticks
Limited fruit, nuts and seeds

FAST FOOD WEEK

Some weeks call for quick fixes and speedy suppers. Often, this can be where diets fail – it can seem quicker and easier to grab something on the go. But being in a rush is no reason to sabotage your weight loss. Here, we have put together a week of fast food, Mount Athos Diet-style, with dishes that can be prepared in 30 minutes or less.

Sunday Breakfast:
Greek Yogurt with Granola and Fruit (page 191)

Sunday Lunch:
Mackerel Salad (page 195)

Sunday Supper:
Spaghetti with Leeks and Butternut Squash (page 205)

Monday Breakfast:
Banana Toast (page 135)

Monday Lunch:
Carrot and Cumin Soup (page 148)

Monday Supper:
Peppers Piedmontese (page 175)
Broccoli with Chilli (page 182)

Tuesday Breakfast:
Bircher Muesli Breakfast Pot (page 187)

Tuesday Lunch:
Greek Salad (page 194)

Tuesday Supper:
Grilled Lemon Salmon (page 211)

Wednesday Breakfast:
Muesli with Fruit Juice (page 139)

Wednesday Lunch:
Avocado Toast (page 181)

Wednesday Supper:
Japanese Noodle Soup (page 149)

Thursday Breakfast:
Banana and Blueberry Smoothie (page 190)

Thursday Lunch:
Egg Fried Rice (page 215)

Thursday Supper:
Pasta with Rocket (page 210)

Friday Breakfast:
Full Greek Breakfast (page 137)

Friday Lunch:
Quick Quinoa Pilaf (page 174)

Friday Supper:
Pea Soup (page 150)
Roast Pepper, Spinach and Orange Salad (page 142)

VEGETARIAN WEEK

Sunday (Moderation Day)
Breakfast
Huevos Rancheros (page 188)
To drink:
- Tea or coffee, small amount of milk
- Small glass of fruit juice

Lunch
Sri Lankan Sweet Potato Soup (page 197)
Serve with:
- Small piece of bread
To drink:
- Herbal tea
- Water or a small glass of fruit juice

Supper
Vegetable Tagine (page 165)
Serve with:
- Small amount of couscous or bulgur wheat, salad or green vegetable
To drink:
- 2 small glasses of red wine
- Water

To follow
Melon with Rosewater (page 218)
1 square of dark chocolate or other small treat

Snacks
Unlimited vegetable sticks
Limited fruit, nuts and seeds
Limited crackers or breadsticks

Monday (Fast Day)

Breakfast

Porridge (page 136)

Serve with:

- Sliced banana

To drink:

- Black tea or coffee/herbal tea
- Water

Lunch

Tuscan Bean Soup (page 146)

Serve with:

- Small amount of wholemeal bread (no butter)

To drink:

- Herbal tea
- Water or a small glass of fruit juice

Supper

Lentil Dal (page 170)

Cauliflower 'Rice' (page 177)

Serve with:

- Indian Salad (page 144)
- Small Indian bread, such as a chapatti

To drink:

- Herbal tea
- Water or a small glass of fruit juice

Snacks

Unlimited vegetable sticks

Limited fruit, nuts and seeds

Tuesday (Moderation Day)
Breakfast
Scrambled Egg with Rye Toast (page 189)
Serve with:
- Fresh or grilled tomatoes

To drink:
- Tea or coffee, small amount of milk
- Small glass of fruit juice

Lunch
Egg Fried Rice (page 215)
To drink:
- Herbal tea
- Water or a small glass of fruit juice

Supper
Baked Sweet Potatoes with Olives and Feta (page 214)
Serve with:
- Large green salad and fresh tomatoes

To drink:
- 2 small glasses of red wine
- Water

To follow
Orange with Mint and Orange Blossom Water (page 219)
1 square of dark chocolate or other small treat

Snacks
Unlimited vegetable sticks
Limited fruit, nuts and seeds
Limited crackers or breadsticks

Wednesday (Fast Day)

Breakfast

Banana Toast (page 135)

To drink:

- Black tea or coffee/herbal tea
- Water

Lunch

Mount Athos White Bean Salad (page 143)

Serve with:

- Large green salad and fresh tomatoes
- Small amount of wholemeal bread (no butter)

To drink:

- Herbal tea
- Water or a small glass of fruit juice

Supper

Moroccan Chickpea and Squash Stew (page 161)

Serve with:

- Small amount of couscous or bulgur wheat, salad or green vegetables

To drink:

- Herbal tea
- Water or a small glass of fruit juice

Snacks

Unlimited vegetable sticks
Limited fruit, nuts and seeds

Thursday (Moderation Day)
Breakfast
Poached Eggs (page 193)
Serve with:
- Rye toast and fresh or grilled tomatoes

To drink:
- Tea or coffee, small amount of milk
- Small glass of fruit juice

Lunch
Hearty Harissa Salad with Greek Yogurt Dressing (page 140)
Serve with:
- Toasted pitta bread

To drink:
- Herbal tea
- Water or a small glass of fruit juice

Supper
Spaghetti with Leeks and Butternut Squash (page 205)
To drink:
- 2 small glasses of red wine
- Water

To follow
Banana 'Ice Cream' (page 220)
1 square of dark chocolate or other small treat

Snacks
Unlimited vegetable sticks
Limited fruit, nuts and seeds
Limited crackers or breadsticks

Friday (Fast Day)
Breakfast
Muesli with Fruit Juice (page 139)
To drink:
- Black tea or coffee/herbal tea
- Water

Lunch
Butternut Squash Soup (page 156)
Serve with:
- Wholemeal roll or small slice of bread
To drink:
- Herbal tea
- Water or a small glass of fruit juice

Supper
Braised Puy Lentils with Bay Leaves (page 172)
Serve with:
- White Bean Mash (page 180), carrots and greens, such as cabbage, chard or kale
To drink:
- Herbal tea
- Water or a small glass of fruit juice

Snacks
Unlimited vegetable sticks
Limited fruit, nuts and seeds

WORKING WEEK

If you work away from home Monday to Friday in an office, factory or shop, diets can often seem a little limited. Not so the Mount Athos Diet. The range of recipes available to eat across the different days make for a truly interesting menu, one that can be easily accommodated via a packed lunch or through the use of a limited workplace kitchen. Equally, the selections below would work well on a picnic.

All the Mount Athos Diet soups can be made portable using a flask to keep them hot until lunchtime, or by the use of a microwave. You will notice we haven't included many sandwich options in the recipe sections, so here you will find more in the way of traditional on-the-go lunches.

Monday
Avocado salad sandwiches
Fresh fruit

Tuesday
Leftover roast chicken made into sandwiches or a salad with plenty of shredded lettuce, salt and pepper, lemon juice/ Greek yogurt

Wednesday
Hummus sandwiches or on toast, with sprouted seeds and slices of fresh tomato

Thursday
Hard-boiled egg with Greek Salad (page 194)

Friday
Black Bean Chilli wrap with salad (page 163)

DINNER PARTY

It's even possible to cater for an entire dinner party using the Mount Athos Diet recipes, with none of your guests knowing that the food you serve is healthy and diet-friendly, this meal won't scupper your weight loss. The following menu is designed to be perfect for a Moderation Day.

When guests arrive:
- Butternut Squash and Rosewater Dip, served with crudités (page 185)
- Pumpkin Seeds with Soy Sauce (page 184)
- Avocado Toasts (made individually in bite-sized portions) (page 181)

To start:
Tuscan Bean Soup with shavings of Parmesan (page 146)
Serve with:
- Warm, crusty bread

Main course:
Poached Salmon with Fennel (page 209)
White Bean Mash (page 180)
French Lettuce, Peas and Mint (page 176)

Dessert:
Pineapple, berry, mint and honey fruit salad
Dark chocolate

To drink:
- Red wine

- Sparkling water with lemon/lime slices or strips of cucumber and plenty of ice
- Coffee

WINTER WARMER MENU

With plenty of warming, spicy dishes on offer, the Mount Athos Diet is full of meals ideal for the colder months. Here is a selection of our favourite winter warmers, and all adhering to the Mount Athos Diet eating plan.

Sunday Breakfast
Huevos Rancheros (page 188)

Sunday Lunch
Sri Lankan Sweet Potato Soup (page 197)

Sunday Supper
Tunisian Fish Tagine (page 200)

Monday Breakfast
Porridge (page 136)

Monday Lunch
Japanese Noodle Soup (page 149)

Monday Supper
Black Bean Chilli (page 163)

Tuesday Breakfast
Banana Pancakes (page 192)

Tuesday Lunch
Butternut Squash Soup (page 156)

Tuesday Supper
Asian Poached Chicken with Sesame Green Beans and jacket potato (page 203)

Wednesday Breakfast
Full Greek Breakfast (page 137)

Wednesday Lunch
Pea Soup (page 150)

Wednesday Supper
Braised Puy Lentils with Bay Leaves (page 172)

Thursday Breakfast
Poached Eggs on rye toast (page 193)

Thursday Lunch
Mackerel Salad (page 195)

Thursday Supper
Spaghetti Arrabiatta (page 160)

Friday Breakfast
Banana Toast (page 135)

Friday Lunch
Moroccan Carrot and Chickpea Soup (page 145)

Friday Supper
Lentil Dal with Cauliflower 'Rice' (pages 170 and 177)

CHAPTER 21

MOUNT ATHOS DIET SUCCESS STORIES

The authors of the Mount Athos Diet were the first three dieters to adopt the eating patterns of the Mount Athos monks, and saw success with their weight-loss journeys. Here are their stories, which explain how each author approached the diet in the context of their own particular circumstances.

RICHARD'S STORY

I decided to properly road test the Mount Athos Diet after a particularly indulgent holiday. After four weeks of serious eating and drinking, with little time for proper exercise, I returned home 3.6 kg (8 lb) heavier than when I'd set off. Even if I lost that weight, I'd still be at least a stone (6.4 kg) heavier than my preferred weight. Something needed to be done.

I set myself a tough target: from 86 kg (193 lb) to 76 kg (168 lb) in 12 weeks – around 0.9 kg (2 lb) a week. I realised that I couldn't achieve this weight loss by dieting alone and that regular, serious exercise would have to be part of the equation. So, not being a fan of gyms or bossy boot camps, I decided that walking would help shift the weight. I live in a city, so country walks would be a rarity; pavement pounding was to be the name of the game. I logged my daily walking distances and over the three months I walked a total of 359 km (223 miles), or nearly 4 km (2½ miles) a day which took me only 45 minutes a day.

The diet itself also helped me shift the required weight within the target time. As my daily walks became a habit, so too did the Mount Athos Diet. In no time I was automatically avoiding all the 'wrong' foods. I was eating differently and drinking less and overall found that monthly food and drink bills fell dramatically.

Some weeks into the diet, I went to a friend's for lunch and was offered a plate of cold meats – ham, beef, salami, chorizo, sausages and so on. I looked at it with alarm; I hadn't touched any processed meats since I started the diet and found the sight quite disturbing. The thing was: I hadn't missed any of the foods I used to enjoy – red meat, sausages, pies, etc. What I had come to enjoy was vegetables (something I had previously eaten out of habit). Also, different ways of cooking chicken and fish. Meals became spicier and tastier. My style of cooking altered, too.

During my three-month period on the Mount Athos Diet things had changed. What food I bought, how I cooked it, portion sizes all changed. And now, six months after I started to diet the mind shift has been extraordinary. I still practise the Mount Athos Diet and still walk every day. Weight loss has stabilised and all in all I am pounds better off in both weight and wallet.

SUE'S STORY

I haven't found the need to 'diet' as such during most of my life. Being trained as a dietitian, I always knew where the problems in food and drink lay, so I did my best to eat well.

I'm not overly zealous though. I love food and cooking, and enjoy exploring ingredients, recipes and the food from all over the world. My approach to food is to eat a healthy diet most of the time, so that when I get the opportunities to cook or eat something indulgent and delicious, it won't be an issue.

However, my steady equilibrium all changed when I moved out of London. I had just passed 40 and moved to a more provincial place. Rather than walking everywhere and rushing around as I did in London, I was cycling (at a leisurely pace) or in a car. I also changed from having a regular office job, to working freelance at home. The prospect of this had always worried me. I knew that I would be tempted to snack more if I was at home alone working. At those moments in the working day when you need a short break, and you normally get a drink or have a quick chat with a colleague, at home I would have a drink, and something to eat with it. Nothing significant, but it all adds up. And when combined with less daily activity, I noticed I was putting on weight, slowly but surely.

My weight increased from 59 kg (130 lb) to nearly 65 kg (143 lb). This translates to a BMI of 24.4, which was still a 'healthy' weight for me – just. The weight gain wasn't instantly recognisable. But I could feel it around my stomach and I was shocked at how quickly and easily it seemed to happen now I was older. As I approached 45 I knew it was a situation that I had to nip in the bud. I was at the midlife crossroad where you either decide to actively keep your weight in control, or you don't. If you don't tackle it, then it's a slippery slope towards an increasingly overweight older life. This has happened to both my formerly trim parents. Not only does this make you less mobile in later years, but there are all the health risks that go with being overweight. So for me it was now or never.

When asked to contribute to the Mount Athos Diet I could immediately see the benefits of the simple rules that Richard had developed. I could see how it would appeal to people who enjoy food and cooking, but are also health conscious and think about the consequences of the food choices they make. When I was younger I had been a very principled vegan for several years, so I knew the Fast Days could be tasty and enjoyable. I also knew that it could help people explore cooking with different ingredients, that would in the long run improve what they ate, and whether they stuck at the diet for any length of time or not.

The concept of dividing the week into days of fasting, moderation and feasting makes good sense. It's an easy way of putting the brakes on the everyday excesses of our modern Western diet. Too many foods are available to us, at almost any moment of the day. So if you like food or find it hard to resist a tempting treat, it is very easy to eat more than you need, and in time to become overweight.

Instead of recommending a strict regime of limited calories to lose weight, as I often did with limited success as a dietitian, the Mount Athos way of moderation brings a new set of principles to the way you eat. The diet doesn't make you fixate on calories and count them every day: instead you follow a new pattern of eating. On Fast Days you need to be very strict about what you eat and drink. More variety is introduced on the three Moderation Days, and on the Feast Day you can eat what you please.

I was also really drawn to the ideas and principles in the diet, as they all made sense for reasons over and above those of just losing weight. I like the frugalness of the approach. It seems to resonate with the times we are in and the need to be careful about our greed and excesses on an overpopulated planet. The diet also makes you eat less meat, which is better for the environment, and for your health – it means your sources of protein will be lower in fat and higher in fibre. When I eat meat I buy the best quality I can afford, choosing organic or free range. The Mount Athos Diet reinforces this idea of quality rather than quantity.

So once I was on board with the Mount Athos Diet I was keen to try the diet myself. I had tried to curb my weight gain in a half-hearted, unsuccessful way beforehand, so I was quite amazed at how easily I seemed to lose weight on it. I liked the way that I felt when I followed it too. It feels positive and good for you, and you feel like you are developing long-term good habits.

Combining the diet with exercise was key for me, and then it all seemed quite effortless (first it was dancing and then it was spinning at the gym). In fact it went so well at the beginning that I got a bit too relaxed about following the rules and then I stopped losing weight. But I didn't gain weight, and I was able to pick up the diet again and continue on a downward trajectory. I'm now steady at my target weight of 60 kg (132 lb) (so I've lost 5 kg/11 lb – over half a stone) and I now just eat in a moderate way most days. But if I find I have put on a bit of weight for some reason, like after a holiday or celebration, I just use a few Fast Days to get my weight back to my new norm. The Mount Athos Diet is a great strategy for getting to a healthy weight and staying there.

LOTTIE'S STORY

Three months after giving birth to my second child in 2010, I weighed myself. I knew I'd be unhappy at the reading on the scales, but I didn't anticipate just how much weight I'd put on during pregnancy and the first weeks and months of parenthood. The scales read 13 st 9 lb (87 kg/192 lb), well above my pre-pregnancy weight of 10 st (64 kg/141 lb) and a BMI of 31.81: officially categorised as obese. I was in shock; I'd put on nearly 4 st (25 kg or 51 lb).

I have always been a food obsessive; working on the BBC Food website, I was surrounded by words, pictures, and conversation about all kinds of exciting foods, and I've always been the sort of person who takes recipe books up to read in bed at night. No TV cookery programme would be missed, and I spent many happy moments wondering how those delicacies on screen might taste. Cooking for friends and family, I would go to painstaking efforts to produce the best food I could cook, often spending the whole day in the kitchen after weeks of planning. So it wouldn't be easy for me to change my habits. After all, the life of a new mum revolves around coffee mornings with other similarly tired and frazzled parents, or playgroups spent stuffing down biscuits and instant coffee in while the kids play. Having little energy due to broken nights didn't help, either. There's no way I could have managed a drastic diet or punishing exercise regime.

I knew things had to change, but I didn't know what to do. And, as a self-confessed greedy foodie, I didn't want to give up all the foods I loved. When I heard about the Mount Athos Diet it seemed like an interesting proposal – break up the week and diet when it was convenient while continuing to enjoy my favourite foods one day a week.

As the weeks went on, I came to understand the framework of the Mount Athos Diet by using a financial budgeting analogy. Before, I'd been eating whatever I liked: effectively maxing out my credit card every day, not caring what I spent or what repercussions I'd have to face further down the line. Now, I could work out what the week had in store and 'spend' accordingly. The balanced, measured approach afforded by the Mount Athos Diet worked well for me. In the space of a year I'd dropped 2½ stone (15 kg/33 lb), moving out of that obese BMI category and feeling much better about myself. My back and knees felt better, relieved of some of the strain they'd been under at my highest weight. By then, my total loss matched the weight of my toddler and, as I carried him up the stairs, I began to see clearly quite how much excess weight I'd been submitting my body to and what damage I must've been doing.

For me, one of the main benefits of the Mount Athos Diet is its flexibility. Always go out with friends on a Tuesday, for drinks and a curry? Make that your Feast Day. Make the diet work for you and your life. That way, you will be more likely to stick to it and see the results you want.

Once the authors had successfully lost weight with the Mount Athos Diet, others joined in and saw similar successes. Read their stories in these testimonials.

DEBBIE'S STORY

I have been dieting since I was teenager. I've tried every diet you can think of: Weight Watchers, Slimming World, G.I., Dukan plus loads of diets from magazines. All of them, in different ways, forced me to eat things that I don't want to eat, such as ready-made meals. These diets were not designed for anyone who wants to cook for themselves; they weren't sensitive to the fact that many people enjoy cooking. Then there was all the calorie counting. In short, I had to stick to their regime that forced me down a pre-conceived path which I was supposed rigorously to follow. You had to stick to all the rules and regulations – and there were always a lot of them.

Lately, I felt that I had arrived at a point in my life where I needed to find a diet that I could stick to and one which wouldn't interfere with my love of cooking. Also, I had some health issues, such as a heart murmur and problems with my joints. I felt that I had to stop all this crazy dieting and find something that I could fit into my life. What appealed to me about the Mount Athos Diet was its flexibility: if I ate something 'fattening', such as cheese or bread, then I could immediately balance it out the following day. I found that I was in charge and could manipulate the diet in order to make it fit into my life style. It's very important that a diet, to be successful and long term, fits into your lifestyle, not the other way round.

I started the Mount Athos Diet about three months ago and so far have lost 10 kg (21 lb). During that period I have been away three times, have had to put it on hold, and then returned to the diet. I'm very pleased with my progress and never felt guilty if I strayed off the path while I was away because I knew that I could always pick up where I left off. My weight didn't increase when I was away, it only stabilised, then continued to drop once I was back home and on the Mount Athos Diet once more.

I know now that I will never go on another diet. If I put any weight back on, I'll just be a little stricter with myself. Real life can get in the way of the most dedicated dieter – parties, going out to a restaurant, being a guest in someone else's home. I explain that I am on a diet and ask for a smaller portion, and I eat very slowly. I know when I've overeaten and then I go on a very strict Fast Day. I'm really getting to like the vegetarian side of the diet and I no longer mind about eating far less meat.

The Mount Athos Diet has altered the way in which I regard food. I can easily eat fish three or four days a week. I've always been wary of beef, even before BSE, and chicken is a good alternative for when I have visitors who are dedicated carnivores.

I now enjoy my food more by concentrating and by putting my knife and fork down while I am eating. It slows my eating down and I chew better. I'm back into all the clothes I haven't been able to wear. The diet has not only altered my shape, it has made me become much more physically active. With my heart murmur I used to become quite scared when I had to puff and pant my way up hills. I feel so much fitter and have much more energy than I've had for a long time. And I no longer have any problems with my joints. I've saved money, too, as meat and dairy products cost a lot of money nowadays.

The Mount Athos Diet is essentially a Mediterranean diet and brings to mind fresh fruit and vegetables. It also has a sunny, light feel to it as opposed to a Northern European diet which is redolent of dumplings and cakes and seriously fattening foods.

ALICE'S STORY

When I began the Mount Athos Diet I was looking for a good way to kick-start a new eating regime. I am a self-confessed foodie and the thought of most diets leaves me depressed as they rarely allow for hearty, good-tasting food.

Once I learnt the 'rules' and retrained my way of eating, the Mount Athos Diet actually freed me from my more destructive eating habits (chocolate is my weakness) and made cooking and eating enjoyable and guilt-free. Alongside the diet I exercised three or four times a week. I lost 4 kg (8 lb) in just two weeks.

The Mount Athos Diet has enough guidelines to keep me on the straight and narrow, but allows room for me to enjoy cooking and eating.

SUSAN'S STORY

I was very slim when I was younger; I weighed about seven and a half stone (48 kg/99 lb). My mother was a terrible cook so I was not interested in food. I met my husband in my early twenties and he is a very good cook. So that's when I really became interested in food and, at the same time, discovered the delights of wine. When I reached my thirties, having had two children, I discovered that I was a stone and a half (9.5 kg/21 lb) over my usual weight. This was not how I saw myself in my head; it is an important thing – how you visualise yourself compared with how you really are.

I followed various fad diets such as the Grapefruit Diet only to find that by the time I had reached my forties I had put on even more weight. By now I was nudging 10½ stone (67 kg/148 lb). So I went on the Slim Fast diet and lost nearly 2 stone (13 kg/29 lb). 'This is great,' I thought. 'Any time I put on weight I can just go back on "the powders".' However, once I had lost the weight I was disinclined to go back on the same old diet. I'd been there and done it before; now it had lost its challenge and had become really boring. Also, a friend yo-yos on this type of diet, her weight at any one time varying by up to 3 stone (19 kg/42 lb). I don't think this is a very healthy approach to weight loss.

Recently, I returned from a long holiday weighing more than I ever had. Something had to be done. I was attracted to the Mount Athos Diet – more a way of eating than the normal, very proscriptive diets. At last, a way of getting the weight off and keeping it off through a very sensible plan. I am quite happy with the Fast Days because I love fruit, and adore the vegetable tagines and curries and stuffed peppers. I start the day with porridge and some bran and wheat germ, with a teaspoon of honey. Then it's often home-made soup for lunch. The diet is so flexible it presents no hardship at all. Also, I have started going to the gym regularly, which is my preferred form of exercise.

When I started on the Mount Athos Diet I was 11 stone 5 lb (70 kg/154 lb); now I'm down to 10 stone 2 lb (67 kg/148 lb). I'm losing weight at a steady 0.9–1.4 kg (2–3 lb) a week. I want to lose another 3 kg (7 lb). At that point I'll stay on the diet, probably dropping to two Fast Days a week, rather than three. If weight looks as if it's returning, I'll simply up the number of Fast Days, cutting out dairy produce and wine, which is very easy to do.

GARY AND SARAH'S STORY

We have both found the basic premise of the Mount Athos Diet easy. The recipes and ideas for how to create filling and tasty meals have been easy to follow, and our habits have changed. We now have very few desserts and have found that the increased intake of veggies is really altogether satisfying.

As an American married couple living in the South of France, the social expectations of summer in France could have been a slight hindrance. With the summer social season of long weekend lunches and similar dinners, fuelled by copious amounts of wine, we feel it's been a victory to hold our own against this tide of French eating and drinking. Our weight has remained steady but our condition and shape has improved measurably. I need the next belt loop now to keep my trousers up.

Doing some form of exercise (something as easy as walking) is a key component to getting the overall effect. For the two of us it was the idea that we weren't trying a severe diet, which we would probably break anyway, but something that made sense and could be followed indefinitely. We will continue.

MARIA'S STORY

I have been on so many diets since my teenage years and battled with my weight, from Weight Watchers to Slimming World, Atkins to Raw Energy.

Last year, at the age of 44, I decided never to diet again and to try not to weigh myself as I am of the belief dieting itself can make you overweight. However, I did decide to try the Mount Athos Diet because for me it didn't feel like a restrictive diet but more in line with what I was starting to do already – to create a sustainable way of eating for the rest of my life.

Having read obsessively about dieting and comfort eating, the one thing that seems so obvious and yet no diets address is the psychological effect of eating. There is a huge amount of guilt associated with eating the 'wrong' food if you are dieting, and there are many reasons someone may eat aside from hunger, emotional eating being a prime example. I think that these issues should be addressed before trying to change or control our eating patterns.

I haven't stuck rigidly to the Mount Athos Diet but I do feel it is building the foundation for a long-term way of living and eating. It fits with my ideal of reducing/eliminating red meat, trying not to eat too much processed or sugary food and not consuming too much alcohol. All of which help me maintain a more even emotional level than the ups and downs I was experiencing from overconsumption. The rate and quality of meat consumption by Western society is not sustainable for our health or the environment so there are many reasons to include vegetarian dishes in your weekly diet. The Mount Athos Diet is great in that respect, as I love cooking with fresh spices. I have also found that snacking on a few nuts instead of reaching for the biscuits has helped keep energy levels up.

Over all I've lost 3 kg (6 lb) in the first month; however, what is more important for me is that I feel more healthy and fitter, my weight is levelling and not bouncing up and down, which means that when I continue to lose weight on the diet it is more likely to last. I am also more inclined to listen to my body now and eat what I need, not for the sake of it or craving rich food.

SUE AND ROBIN'S STORY

We recently bought new scales and had a nasty shock – it turned out that we were both 3 kg (7 lb) heavier than we had thought. We have friends who regularly go on the Cabbage Soup diet, but of course once they come off it, the weight piles on again. We had no intention of letting that happen to us.

On the Fast Days we have really enjoyed rediscovering porridge. It is delicious with a spoonful of honey, half a banana and almond milk. Then for lunch we'll generally have home-made soup – hearty and chunky made from all those odd veggies that we find in the fridge. These are so easy to make. Sometimes we'll keep the soup for evening to enjoy with a slice of bread – without butter, though. We use hummus as a replacement. For our evening meals we might have spicy veggie dishes, curries, dal, that kind of thing. Sometimes, for simplicity, we go for baked beans on a baked potato. What is less easy for us is no alcohol on the Fast Days, but even so we have soon adapted to it and it no longer represents a problem. Giving up dairy for three days a week is really good for us, too.

Since starting on the diet I went away for 10 days and even though I was no longer in charge of what I cooked I found that I'd gone off meat, preferring fish dishes. I no longer buy crisps, ready-meals or processed meats. Last night we had tuna with some chopped up anchovies and a mixed bean salad – really tasty. The Mount Athos Diet has definitely changed our way of eating. There are so many foods out there, which are plentiful and good for you, and it is not necessary to rely on super-market ready-meals or takeaways.

We also exercise. We have a dog that needs walking every day, so we get out of the house. Robin is joining the local gym and is determined to carry on and lose a stone (6.4 kg/14 lb) over the next four months. He plans to go at 7pm, which for Robin is normally a dangerous time, as he does like his regular glass of beer and dish of peanuts.

EUGENIE'S STORY

My mum was always on and off different diets for most of her life, and I didn't want to do that. It's not good for your weight to yo-yo like that. So I'd never followed a diet before. I've put on a bit of weight as I've got older though, so I thought I would try this diet as it seemed simple and not a silly fad diet. But it also wasn't just the usual and obvious healthy eating advice.

In my anti-diet spirit, I didn't weigh myself, but I was amazed at how my waistline got slimmer after following the diet. Trousers that were getting tight are now loose. The diet really changes the way you eat in the long run; it makes you more aware of what you are eating and helps you make better choices. We always had meat and two veg every day, but now we're eating less meat, and it's really helped to break my bad habits of having too much sugar and sweets. I was rarely hungry on the diet, only the first few evenings.

After just one week, I found it was an easy rhythm to follow. It's easy to get in a rut with the way you eat, and I think I'd been eating the same things for many years. The diet really helped me to change the way I eat and I actually enjoyed the challenge of finding new things to eat on Fast Days.

AFTER THE
MOUNT ATHOS DIET
– WHAT THEN?

Once upon a time there was a man and wife. They had achieved many of their ambitions in life, but one important goal remained outstanding. They wanted to swim to Japan.

They discussed this and one day set off. Not practised swimmers, at first they found it difficult. They were aware of how heavy their limbs felt. They ached with the constant effort, especially when the current was against them. Gradually, however, their bodies got used to swimming and they developed a style that became effortless and rhythmical. They learnt how to find food in the water, how to nourish themselves and how to use their bodies effortlessly.

Their senses became more attuned to the water around them, and how it changed colour as the days went by. And they became aware of the creatures in the water; the small silver fish that swam with them; the dark shadows that skimmed by them in the deep. They became aware of how the sound of the waves changed as they lapped their ears, and they felt the subtle changes of the weather as breezes turned into winds and died down again. They developed a refined sense of smell and could detect tiny changes in the environment by the scent carried to them on the breeze.

They swam for days and weeks with no sign of land on the horizon. They swam on and on until one morning they recognised the shoreline of Japan. As they approached they became quiet and eventually they knew. At that moment, they turned back to the sea and swam on.

CONVERSION TABLES

Metric to imperial conversions are close approximations. Never mix metric with imperial, or vice versa, when cooking.

Spoon measurements given in our recipes are always level, unless otherwise specified.

WEIGHT

Metric	Approx. Imperial
25 g	1 oz
50 g	2 oz
75 g	3 oz
100–125 g	4 oz
150 g	5 oz
175 g	6 oz
200g	7 oz
225g	8 oz
250 g	9 oz
275 g	10 oz
300 g	11 oz
325–350 g	12 oz
375 g	13 oz
400 g	14 oz

425 g	15 oz
450 g	16 oz (1 lb)
500 g (½ kg)	17.5 oz
1 kg	2.2 lb

LIQUID VOLUME

Metric	Approx. Imperial
25 ml	1 fl oz
50 ml	2 fl oz
100 ml	4 fl oz
150 ml	5 fl oz
300 ml	10 fl oz
600 ml	20 fl oz (1 pint)
1000 ml (1 litre)	35 fl oz

OVEN TEMPERATURES

140°C	275°F	Gas mark 1
150°	300°	2
170°	325°	3
180°	350°	4
190°	375°	5
200°	400°	6
220°	425°	7
230°	450°	8
240°	475°	9

APPENDIX II

FURTHER SOURCES AND RESOURCES

COOKERY BOOKS

The Cuisine of the Holy Mountain Athos by Monk Epiphanios of Mylopotamos (Synchroni Orizontes, Greece)

Greek Monastery Cooking by Archimandrite Dositheos (St Nectarios Press, 2003)

The Complete Book of Greek Cooking – the recipe club of St. Paul's Greek Orthodox Cathedral (HarperPerennial, USA, 1990)

Vegan Planet by Robin Robertson (The Harvard Common Press, USA, 2003)

Vefa's Kitchen by Vefa Alexiadou (Phaidon, 2009)

OTHER BOOKS

Mount Athos: Renewal in Paradise by Graham Speake (New Haven Connecticut & London: Yale University Press, 2002)

Pantokrator: an introduction to Orthodoxy by Trevor Curnow (Cambridge Scholars Publishing, 2007)

Yoga as Medicine by Timothy McCall M.D. (Bantam Dell N.Y. 2007)

Wherever You Go, There You Are: mindfulness meditation for everyday life by Jon Kabat-Zinn (Piatkus Books Ltd., 2013 edition)

INTERNET LINKS

The *Friends of Mount Athos* online:
The Society of the Friends of Mount Athos is dedicated to the study and promulgation of knowledge of the history, culture, arts, architecture, natural history and literature of the Orthodox monasteries of Mount Athos, and to the promotion of the religious and other charitable work of the Holy Community and the monasteries, both those located on Mount Athos, and those elsewhere which are dependent or connected in some way with Mount Athos. www.athosfriends.org

Calculate your healthy weight with the online NHS calculator: www.nhs.uk/tools/pages/healthyweightcalculator.aspx?WT. mc_id=101007
or download their free BMI calculator app (for iPhone or iPad) at: www.nhs.uk/Tools/Pages/BMI-iPhone-app.aspx

Also for further reading, recipes and Mount Athos monastery products: www.pemptousia.com and www.monastiriaka.gr

Two must-see videos about life on the Holy Mountain:
  CNN: 60 Minutes documentary – Part One
  http://www.youtube.com/watch?v=WFW8lHfwAdo
  Part Two
  http://www.youtube.com/watch?v=J1lvruy-j2c

SOURCES OF WINES FROM MOUNT ATHOS

Monoxilitis
63075 Ouranoupoli, P.O. Box 2084, Greece
Tel: +30 23770 21136
www.monoxilitis.com
e-mail: shop@monoxilitis.com

Tsantali
Agios Pavlos, 63080 Halkidiki, Greece
Tel: +30 23990 76100
Their red wine, a Cabernet Sauvignon, is available from major
Waitrose stores throughout the UK.

www.monastiriaka.gr
See their website for wines from the Holy Monasteries of Vato-
pedi (Syrah, Cabernet Sauvignon) and Simonos Petras.

www.drinkaware.co.uk

ENDNOTES

Chapter 7: Getting Prepared For The Diet

[1] http://www.nhs.uk/chq/Pages/3215.aspx?CategoryID=52

Chapter 8: Tips For Achieving Success

[1] Muckelbauer, Rebecca, et al. 'Association between water consumption and body weight outcomes: a systematic review.' *The American Journal of Clinical Nutrition* 98.2 (2013): 282–299.

[2] Swithers, Susan E. 'Artificial sweeteners produce the counterintuitive effect of inducing metabolic derangements.' *Trends in Endocrinology & Metabolism* (2013).

[3] Rolls, Barbara J., Elizabeth A. Bell, and Michelle L. Thorwart. 'Water incorporated into a food but not served with a food decreases energy intake in lean women.' *The American Journal of Clinical Nutrition* 70.4 (1999): 448–455.

ACKNOWLEDGEMENTS

This book is the result of a collaborative effort, requiring the knowledge of three authors, the assistance of two editors, the input from a team of voluntary dieters and recipe testers, and the forbearing patience of our families.

Our grateful thanks go to Louise Francis, our initial commissioning editor at Ebury Publishing, whose early foresight, enthusiasm and encouragement saw the project off the ground. More recently, we have worked closely with her successor Sam Jackson, a woman whose sharp intellectual discipline and instructive comments have helped us to refine, rewrite and polish key sections of the book. Our eagle-eyed copyeditor Kathy Steer's professional advice has been of great help in reworking the final manuscript.

The success stories of an army of voluntary dieters have added a valuable dimension to the development of the Mount Athos Diet. Our grateful thanks go to: Maria Bowers, Mary and Courtney Goff (USA), Alice Hendy, Debbie Kolombos, Sarah and Gary Legon (France), Eugenie Manders, Susan Oatley, Sue and Robin Parker, and many others whose input has been invaluable.

Thank you to Dave Lewis and Lucy Rees of Bristol Bootcamp Company for their advice and encouragement, and to the team at Riverford Organic Farms and to Reg the Veg, Clifton, Bristol for supplying beautiful vegetables for use in recipe development.

We appreciate Sue Knight's kind permission to use 'Swimming to Japan', reproduced from her exemplary book, *NLP at Work*.

Finally, our thanks to John Arnell, who has shown generous support, interest and belief in the book.

A proportion of author proceeds of this book will go to the Friends of Mount Athos. The objectives of the society include the study and knowledge of the history, culture, arts, architecture, natural history and literature of the Orthodox monasteries of Mount Athos, and the promotion of the religious and other charitable work of the Holy Community and monasteries of Mount Athos.

INDEX